Extraordinary Vessels

Kiiko Matsumoto

Stephen Birch

Paradigm Publications Brookline, Massachusetts

1986

Extraordinary Vessels

Kiiko Matsumoto
Stephen Birch

ISBN 0-912111-35-6

Library of Congress Cataloging-in-Publication Data
Matsumoto, Kiiko.
Extraordinary Vessels

Includes index.
1. Acupuncture. I. Birch, Stephen. II Title.
{DNLM: 1. Acupuncture. WB 369 M4335e}
RM184 M376 615.8'92 86–5069
ISBN 0-912111-35-6

This book was produced and typeset using software provided by Textware International of Cambridge, Massachusetts; the UNIX operating system developed by Bell Laboratories; and software developed by Redwing Book Company.

Published by
Paradigm Publications
44 Linden Street
Brookline, Massachusetts 02146

Editors: Robert L. Felt, Martha Lee Fielding
Cover design: Cardinal Graphics
Illustrations: Herb Rich III

10 9 8 7

Dedication

We dedicate this book to Sohichiro and Yuichiro Tobe of Ido No Nippon Sha for their generosity and commitment to Oriental medicine. We further dedicate this text to Drs. Tsugio Nagatomo, Yoshio Manaka, Osamu Ito, Michi Tokito and Naoichi Kuzome for their tireless dedication and creative contributions to the knowledge and development of Oriental medicine.

Acknowledgements

I thank Yuichiro Tobe for making so much available to me: books, papers, reports, printed characters and information. My special thanks go to my teachers who gave so many hours to my education. There are many to whom I can only offer my most profound gratitude: Tsugio Nagatomo, the founder of the "plus-minus" needle system; Yoshio Manaka, a modern father of Oriental medicine, inventor of the ion cords and ion beam generator, the Manaka hammer technique and the teacher from whom I have received immense intellectual stimulation; Osamu Ito, specialist in extraordinary meridian magnetic therapies; Ichiro Iwata, a classmate who introduced me to Michi Tokito; Michi Tokito, who discovered the extraordinary vessel pulse diagnosis and treatment system; Naoichi Kuzome, who taught me the essence of abdominal diagnosis. Finally, without the influence of Shigehisa Kuriyama, whose work will lead the advance of sinology in the generation to follow Joseph Needham, this book would have been considerably more difficult.

It is a great pleasure and privilege to introduce these teachers and their work to the West. Their research into the claims of Chinese medicine is the direct continuation of the insightful curiosity and will to heal that is the deepest tradition of Chinese medicine. Our appreciation of the ancient healers of China who left their wonderful treatment styles as a gift for us today must be boundless. There remain many materials and styles that are unknown to the West, the extraordinary vessels among them. I hope that some of the readers of this book will continue this research.

Kiiko Matsumoto
Boston, Massachusetts
April, 1986

Acknowledgements

I would like to thank my family, and particularly my mother and my sister Helen, for their patience and understanding. I am deeply indebted to Dr. Yoshio Manaka for his kindness and encouragement, to Jim Oschman, PhD. for his generosity, support and help, and to Bob Felt and Martha Fielding for their friendship, advice and skills. I will always be indebted to the ancient Chinese healers whose insight and genius passed to us the profound theoretical and practical heritage of Oriental medicine in which we may constantly find new ideas and insights for our age.

Stephen Birch
Boston, Massachusetts
April, 1986

Introduction

This book began as two chapters of a larger work started in 1983, tentatively titled *Hara: Reflections on the Sea,* a study of abdominal palpation in acupuncture. When reviewing the final draft, it was evident that much of what was necessary to the understanding of the extraordinary vessels in acupuncture was lacking. Further, understanding the energetics of the extraordinary vessels was a considerable contribution to a practical and theoretical understanding of the role of the hara, the abdomen, in human life. In the Orient the theoretical work and treatment developments of Tsugio Nagatomo, Yoshio Manaka, Osamu Ito, and Michi Tokito have profoundly influenced leading practitioners in China, Japan and Korea. Thus, publication was delayed as this material was further researched for presentation.

As this information was merged with the text, it became apparent that the results would never fit between a single set of covers. Each theoretical discussion, each diagnostic schema, and each treatment system required background information that was not available in English texts. As the project expanded, so too did the new translations and research necessary to present cogent explanations. By late 1985 the written output of the project exceeded 1,200 pages of manuscript draft. At times it appeared that the scope of the project would permanently outpace the ability to research and publish.

What had begun as a brief discussion of extraordinary vessel theory had become pathway descriptions, references to classical treatment modes, and descriptions of modern treatment systems. This expansion, at least in part the result of curiosity, was also driven by the need to support much of the modern thought concerning acupuncture with the classical references from which the ideas evolved. This was particularly true in regard to the extraordinary vessels and the art of palpation. For example, one consistent application of the extraordinary vessels is the correction of structural imbalance, the actual, physical disruptions of the body's symmetry. In clinical practice these present not only as debilitating deformations, but also as sub-clinical differences in limb length, point or area reactivity and sensitivity. Without an understanding of how the extraordinary vessels effect changes in the physical structure of the body, the correspondences that are the basis of the structural treatments appear to be merely reflexive therapy. Without the perspective afforded by later research, the structural orientation of treatments in classics such as the *Zhen Ju Da Cheng* are easily missed. In turn, unless the centrality and depth of extraordinary vessel energetics is considered, their functions are difficult to distinguish.

Thus, this book acquired a separate identity among the documentation prepared for the original text. It has a dual role. First, it is a presentation of the information that has lead to the development of successful treatment systems; and second, it is a pointer toward information that will be published at a later date. As such, it contains some forward references to more detailed discussions that will be continued in association with diagnostic and treatment systems that use the information in this text as part of their theoretical and practical background. However, as a subject of inquiry, the eight vessels are among the most interesting elements of acupuncture theory. Since their first systematic descriptions, they have been associated with the most subtle energetic transformations. The biorhythmic, cosmologic and prenatal qualities ascribed to these vessels are a bridge between some of the most intriguing elements of Oriental philosophy and some of the most effective acupuncture practices.

By virtue of this close association with the cosmological forces described by the Chinese physicians, extraordinary vessel theory also leads us to consider some of the modern, Western explanations of the energies at the roots of life process and physical matter. Certainly, it is an aspect of Oriental medicine rich with possibility, both practical and theoretical, that has produced some of the most fascinating medical thought in the vast history of Chinese medicine. As an introduction to modern treatment styles, annotated with historical details, opinions and variations, we hope this book will provide a useful reference and therapeutic guide for exploring some of the most profound and insightful regions of Oriental medicine.

Table of Contents

Extraordinary Vessels

The Extraordinary Vessels

The eight extraordinary vessels, the *qi jing ba mai* [奇經八脈], constitute a fascinating level of energetic theory and treatment in Chinese medicine. Throughout medical history there have been many different ideas concerning their nature, their pathways, functions, associated symptomology and treatment. Not until the Ming dynasty, when a revolutionary new treatment style developed, had there been any practical consensus regarding these vessels, nor had they been systematically described by reference to the eight "master points."[1] During this period, the famous doctor Li Shi Zhen wrote an entire text devoted to the theory and herbal treatment of extraordinary vessel energetics.[2]

Current clinical practice utilizing the extraordinary vessels demonstrates their vast versatility and effectiveness, and allows us to hypothesize some interesting functions and relationships, both in Oriental medicine and Western science. In this book, we will describe the work of two modern Japanese practitioners who use the eight extraordinary vessels extensively, Ms. Michi Tokito and Mr. Osamu Ito.

In addition, we will describe the theoretical basis of a powerful extraordinary vessel treatment system developed by Dr. Yoshio Manaka of Japan that demonstrates the clinical use of the extraordinary vessels. He has proposed and clinically proven special techniques of stimulating the body's intrinsic bioelectrical systems. These procedures involve the use of "ion-pumping" cords, unidirectional diode connectors, that are capable of directed ion transfer. Dr. Manaka's theories of diagnosis and treatment of the extraordinary vessels are the most coherent available and are more widely applicable than any in the medical literature. His use of the ion pumping cords is a substantial practical justification of his theories. The embryological, biorhythmic, physiological and practical details of Dr. Manaka's ideas and procedures are presented in another text in association with the abdominal palpation system necessary for their use.[3] While it is not entirely clear how influential Dr. Manaka's work has been on the work of practitioners such as Ms. Tokito and Mr. Ito, they do utilize concepts that he helped develop in the 1950's and 1960's. Certainly, it would not be possible to do any serious research or scholarship of the extraordinary vessels without referring to his work and that of his associate Dr. Kazuko Itaya.

Following Dr. Manaka's practice of examining classical ideas and proposing modern clinical uses, tests and theories, our discussions are intended to stimulate and promote scholarship and research. Absolute statements of principle are for matters much smaller and less central than the extraordinary vessels. The purpose of this text is to present the historical background and the essential theoretical and clinical detail necessary for the use of the extraordinary vessels in acupuncture practice. The clinically oriented sections of the text describe the symptomologies of both modern and classical sources.

Terminology

Any acupuncture text must explain some common terminology. We assume familiarity with basic terms such as qi, meridians, acupoints, yin and yang. However, some of the key concepts of this text deserve consideration. Bear in mind that simple, definitive meanings are for smaller ideas. Many, if not most, terms in Oriental medicine have numerous meanings, each of which depends on context. Often, there is no simple English equivalent; attempts to create simple cognates result in gross simplification or misuse of terms in some specific contexts. Meanings have flavor. The flavor of a character is often determined by its etymology.[4] In most instances we have left the specialized terms in romanized form; English readers have demonstrated little difficulty in absorbing such words into their vocabulary. Multiplicity is evident. As is clear in some classical quotations, terms often imply function as much as they imply identity. Different words for the different functions of a single entity are not an unknown occurrence.

The principal exception to the rule of leaving Chinese words in romanized form is the word "extraordinary" itself. The term qi [奇], that we have translated as "extraordinary," generally refers to something exceptional, unusual, strange, rare or wonderful. For instance, it is used to reference the yang, odd numbers. The oldest usage of this term occurs in reference to an unusually shaped or deformed body, someone hunched over, sloping to one side or handicapped by a physical deformity. Such reference to bodily shape or structure is interesting to many practitioners, notably Dr. Manaka and

Mr. Ito, who have found that treatment of the extraordinary vessels is able to correct structural imbalances or deformities. Some of the modern theories of the extraordinary vessels concern their structural and topological qualities.

In English literature we often find the term *qi* of *qi jing ba mai* loosely translated as "extra" or "secondary." These translations imply that these vessels are subordinate to the twelve meridians. This is an unfortunate mistranslation that more accurately reflects the order of teaching acupuncture concepts than it demonstrates the place of the extraordinary vessels in human energetic anatomy. As we will see, the extraordinary vessels are more primary than the twelve meridians. Functionally, they are certainly not simply additional trajectories.

The names of the vessels are also a key to how we think of them. The term *du,* often translated as *governing,* refers to a general, someone who controls. *Ren,* usually translated as "conception," refers to pregnancy, responsibility, or obligation. It can mean "to accept" or "to hold something in front of the abdomen." *Dai* refers to a belt or girdle that acts as a support. *Chong* means a street. It is used to express the idea of passing or transformation. In some contexts chong refers to alchemical transformation, two entities "crashing together" to produce something different. *Qiao* generally means "the heel," or "to stand on the toes." It often indicates the action of the heel rising up; it further means to walk on one's toes with the legs stretched. Most interestingly, it refers to the action of kicking one's foot as high as possible. *Wei* denotes a rope and is often translated as "link," or "bind." Specifically, it refers to a rope that is tied around something, pulling it down and securing it.

Dr. Manaka discovered important clinical rules for the use of the qiao mai and wei mai vessels because of differences in the meaning of the characters. He was able to posit that the wei mai controlled downward movement, while the qiao mai controlled upward movement, because of the "pulling down" and "rising up" connotations of the terms. Through clinical corroboration of this theory, he has determined that it is preferable to treat the wei mai before treating the qiao mai using the ion pumping cords, when there is evidence that the patient's qi is rising. Given the clinical prevalence of "rebellious qi," this is indeed useful.

Historical Review

Three major components comprise the study of the extraordinary vessels: their pathways, the various theories that describe their function and the symptoms and treatments associated with each vessel. The earliest descriptions of the extraordinary vessels concern the pathways. Most, if not all, later commentaries offer variations, additions or opinions concerning the descriptions found in the *Su Wen* and *Ling Shu*. Descriptions of the extraordinary vessels are scattered among many chapters of both the *Ling Shu* and *Su Wen*.[5] When the twelve meridians are described in the *Ling Shu*, the entirety of Chapter 10 is devoted to their pathways. Many of these early discussions contradict each other, intimating that different authors produced different sections. This suggests that the function and use of the extraordinary vessels was not fully developed during the early and middle Han dynasty. Certainly, the ideas were still evolving.

In modern discussions of the extraordinary vessels there is a general consensus regarding their pathways, a result of of the considerable work accomplished in the period bridging the compilation of the *Su Wen* and the arrival of the Ming dynasty. This same evolution is apparent in discussions of symptomology and treatment. There are symptom descriptions in the *Su Wen* and *Ling Shu*, some of which are unclear. The *Nan Jing*, an important early acupuncture text and a major commentary and expansion of the *Su Wen* and *Ling Shu*, written circa 100 BC to 100 AD, systematized and simplified both the pathways and symptomology. Clearly the author of the *Nan Jing* was a clinician of considerable skill. In his work there was a constant attempt to cut through the theoretical knots of the earlier books; the descriptions of both pathways and symptoms were concise. Ironically, as is the case with many great clinicians, the treatment descriptions were neither complete nor systematic.

Some description of pulse types associated with each of the extraordinary vessels was given by Wang Shu He, who wrote the *Mai Jing*, the famous pulse classic,[6] and a major commentary on the *Nan Jing*, circa 300 AD. These representations appear to be the basis of Li Shi Zhen's description of the pulse types for each of the extraordinary vessels.[7] While the descriptions of both Wang Shu He and Li Shi Zhen are evocative and interesting, they are as equally difficult to understand and translate. We have included Wang Shu He's descriptions in this text only as an historical reference. From a practical viewpoint, his descriptions remain somewhat unclear. The theories from the *Nan Jing* and Wang Shu He regarding the extraordinary vessels are the stepping stones between the often obscure and contradictory information in the *Su Wen* and *Ling Shu* and later systematic presentations. In the *Nan Jing* we find a clear development of the energetic theory of the extraordinary vessels. This theory provides a perspective that distinguishes the extraordinary vessels from five element and meridian energetics, and provides us with insight into the nature of the body's energies, the nature of life and the rationale of the treatment procedures associated with these vessels. Wang Shu He had a profound understanding of *Nan Jing*, and contributed greatly to the theories of the extraordinary vessels with his attempts to systematize treatment points, pulse diagnosis and biorhythmic descriptions. These descriptions are rooted in *Nan Jing* energetics.

The author of the *Nan Jing*, though probably not the originator of all these ideas, is nonetheless a powerful protagonist. The enthusiasm with which he champions these ideas has caught the attention of many practitioners and scholars through the centuries. Many Asian commentaries on the *Nan Jing* attempt to clarify these ideas. Most scholars feel that these theories are rooted in Daoist philosophy and contemplative practice.[8] Certainly, many of the concepts may be found in later Daoist literature. If the Daoist influence on the development of extraordinary vessel theory was pervasive, the sparcity of the Han dynasty texts might be explained by the intellectual environment in which they were written. The *Su Wen* and *Ling Shu* descriptions of the extraordinary vessels may have been brief references to Daoist knowledge. Obviously, there is a considerable probability that the ideas were simply at the nascence of their evolution. Although the beginning of a systematic treatment approach could be found in Wang Shu He's commentary, clearly the development was still partial.[9]

The first complete and systematic treatment description of the extraordinary vessels is found in the *Zhen Jiu Da Quan*, written in 1439 AD, wherein the eight master or treatment points are clearly described. By the time of the *Zhen Jiu Da Cheng* in 1601 AD, there was a precise and thorough treatment approach for the extraordinary vessels, following the style established by the earlier *Da Quan* and describing the eight master points, their uses alone, their use in pairs and in combination with other points.

The *Zhen Jiu Da Quan* also made other important contributions. It clearly described a systematic, biorhythmic treatment style based on daily and bihourly stem and branch changes.[10] These biorhythmic treatments are some of the most interesting and useful parts of acupuncture theory and practice. It is impossible to say with certainty that these ideas were developed earlier and transmitted by oral tradition, or were the development of Xu Feng, the author of the *Da Quan*.[11] Whatever the heritage or source, these remarkable theories, positing that the human body is affected by cosmological cycles, have enlarged the idea of environment in Oriental medicine.

Xu Feng described the eight extraordinary vessels with reference to the temporal sequence of the trigrams and to their eight treatment points. These points are usually called "master" points and sometimes "respectable" points.[12]

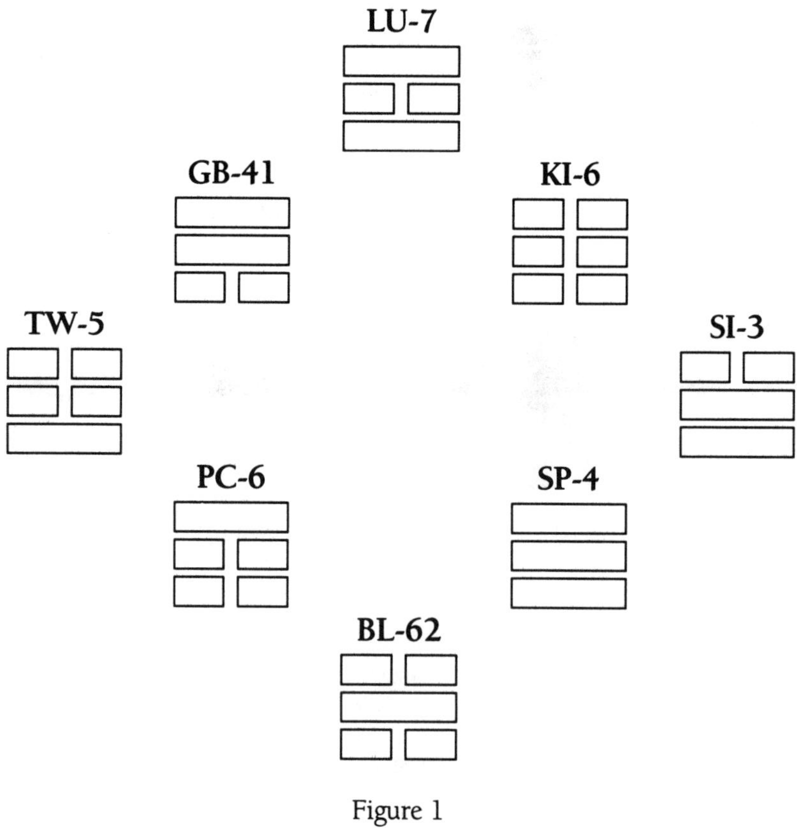

Figure 1

Part of the explanation for these relationships among the extraordinary vessels and the sequence of trigrams is that functionally the eight vessels are four paired sets:[13]

chong mai ◄—► yin wei mai
ren mai ◄—► yin qiao mai
dai mai ◄—► yang wei mai
du mai ◄—► yang qiao mai

These relationships are described further as:[14]

Extraordinary Vessel Relationships			
Point	*Vessel*	*Relation*	*Meeting Places*
SP-4	chong mai	father	heart, chest and stomach
PC-6	yin wei mai	mother	
SI-3	du mai	husband	lateral edges of the bridge of the nose next to the eyes, at the back of the neck, ears, shoulders, arms and the small intestine and bladder meridians
BL-62	yang qiao mai	wife	
GB-41	dai mai	male	the lateral aspect of the eyes, behind the ears, cheeks, neck and shoulders
TW-5	yang wei mai	female	
LU-7	ren mai	master	the "supporter of the lungs" (trachea and bronchi), throat and diaphragm
KI-6	yin qiao mai	guest	

The *Zhen Jiu Da Cheng* also makes interesting comments about the eight vessels as they relate to areas of the body:

> ***The yang qiao, yang wei, du and dai mai mainly treat diseases of the shoulders, back, lumbar and thighs that are superficial. The yin qiao, yin wei, ren and chong mai mainly treat diseases of the heart, abdomen, ribs and sides of the body that are in the lining {inside}.***[15]

The selection of these four pairs of points is probably based on the same point pairing in an earlier text, the *Zhen Jing Zhi Nan, Acupuncture Text South Pointer,* written circa 1295 AD. In this text, SP-4 was paired with PC-6, LU-7 with KI-6, SI-3 with BL-62 and GB-41 with TW-5. However, no clear mention was made of the eight extraordinary vessels in regard to these four pairs of points. The pairs were described as special points, that when treated singly or together would control and cure many disorders.[16] Thus, this text likely influenced Xu Feng's theories.

Many of these developments survive in modern clinical practice. In Dr. Manaka's work, areas where the vessels meet or that may be treated through the extraordinary vessels are often significant diagnostic sites. This is also apparent in the treatment systems described later in this text.

The Nan Jing Theory

The *Nan Jing* extraordinary vessel theory depends on the concept of an energetic center in the body, the "moving qi between the kidneys." In many texts the moving qi is identified with, or related to, ming men, the "small heart" and qihai dantian. The energetic center was known as:

> ***The root of the twelve meridians, fundamental to the five yin and six yang organs;***
> ***the source of the triple warmer, the gate of breathing;***
> ***the source of the vital qi.***[17]

While this center is located in the body, it is also the site of many energetic transformations that reach beyond the body. Ultimately, the source of the center is the heaven—person—earth interaction from which life is generated. Thus, the energies of the center are the essential procreative and generative energies of jing and shen. The energies produced in the center are the main energies of nutrition and protection and the meridian qi. The macrocosmic—microcosmic analogy of Chinese cosmology is completed in the body's center. Just as heaven has a point of origin or energetic center, "tai yi," the great one, so too does the body. The moving qi between the kidneys is the tai yi of the body, the great one from which yin and yang evolve. It is the root and origin of all the body's energetic systems.

In the *Nan Jing* and the Daoist treatises, one concept used to name the origin of human energies within the cosmos was "no-form." The master of the heart, pericardium and the triple warmer have "a name but no form."[18] According to the Daoists, no-form is the "tiny jing" that is the precursor of all material substance.[19] It is the ancestor of matter; it's child is light; it's grandchild is water. All is created from no-form.[20] No-form arises directly from the tai yi, the great one,[21] from which everything else materializes, heaven and earth, yin and yang.[22] No-form creates form, the body, which is continually transformed and animated by shen, sometimes called the spirit.[23]

The traditional Chinese idea of no-form stretches the credulity of those who cannot accept that an ancient society produced powerfully sophisticated ideas. It is clearly interpretable as the universal matrix of energy from which springs all material, animate and inanimate. As it notes the birth of water, the symbol of the ultimate source of matter, from light, energy, it is a direct parallel of modern ideas of the energetic origin of matter. It posits no-form as what we would now call the unifying field. David Bohm's idea of an "implicate order" a "vast ocean of energy" in "space," a vast universal hidden matrix,[24] is much like this ancient cosmological concept.

The transformations of no-form into the energies that are the basis of acupuncture theory occurs in the energetic center, the abdomen, the hara. The triple warmer, master of the heart, pericardium and ming men are the energetic creations of no-form, the first materializations of energy that precede all other material and energetic processes in the body. They function to "step down" the energies of the universe, transforming them to energies that function in the human body. These energies are the center of the body's energetic systems, the first materializations of yin and yang, symbolized as fire and water.[25]

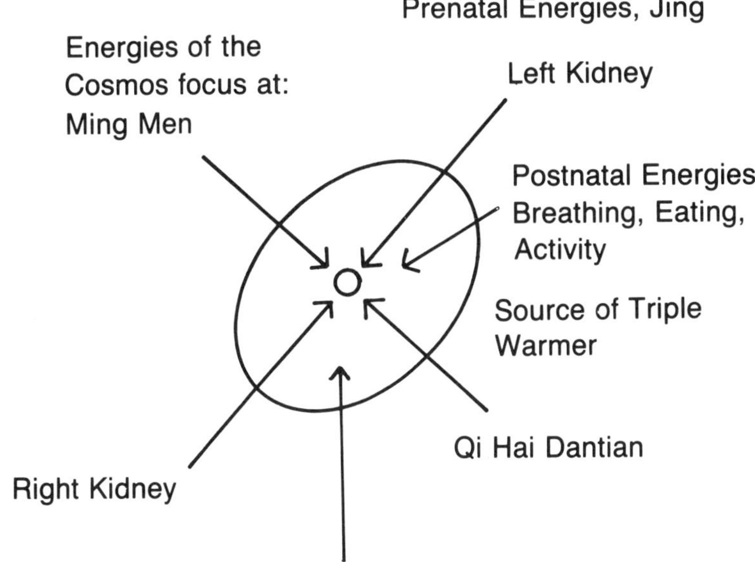

Figure 2 Moving Qi Between the Kidneys

The energies of the cosmic no-form focus at ming men. They project forward to the area of the moving qi. Ming men is related to the master of the heart and pericardium. The triple warmer begins or is centered in the area of the moving qi. Ming men, master of the heart and the triple warmer have an energetic nature closer to no-form and thus transform this cosmic energy and stimulate the moving qi. Here, the prenatal and postnatal energies are transformed. Ming men, master of the heart and the triple warmer support all the body's energetic transformations, including the five element and ten stem relationships, the cycles of the twelve meridians and collaterals and their associated organ systems and functions. All are rooted in the moving qi.

The eight extraordinary vessels are also rooted here, originating at the tai yi, the moving qi. The ren, chong and du mai are frequently described as having their beginning in the uterus. Often, the uterus is equated with the moving qi or described as the site where the moving qi resides. The term we translate here as "uterus" does not refer exclusively to the physical structure, but as well to a set of functions. One conceptual approach may be drawn from considering the embryogenesis of the ren, chong and du mai as they relate to the primordial germ layers of the endoderm, mesoderm and ectoderm.

The chong mai is sometimes identified with the moving qi. The du and ren mai are usually described as the yin—yang branches of the moving qi. The chong and du mai were seen as the "way" of the twelve meridians, responsible for their movement and return to the meeting point at LU-9. Thus, the twelve meridians, the organ systems, the triple warmer system and the extraordinary vessels were each seen to begin at the center. The image emerging from the classical texts is that of a vortex. The cosmic energies come to a point at the center of our being; these energies are the powers of life, the generative force of the universe. From this center the cosmic energies change, transmute, merge and radiate in concentric systems.

The concept is symbolically powerful and complete. Heaven, the archetypical creative, yang force represents the entire set of kinetic energies. Earth, the ultimate yin symbol, is the representative of all that is formative. These cosmological energies pre-exist man, yet are essential to human life. Both meet, focus and are transformed in human life. The physical location of these transformations lies between ming men at the back, and the hara. The more generalized energies take on different aspects as the triple warmer and the master of the heart. In turn, these functions precede and support each of the more specialized energetic systems.

This idea has important therapeutic implications that are the base of the asymptomatic tradition in acupuncture: great physicians treat root problems before attending to local symptoms. Certainly, in both classic and modern treatment sources, distinctions are made between root and local treatments. The model of human energetics just described provides a practical basis for these distinctions. Essentially, problems of the energetic center are root problems. Problems that arise in the branches, the meridians or organs, are symptomatic problems. Problems of the tai yi are given priority in treatment. In Japan, tradition teaches that this may be accomplished at the level of either the five elements or the extraordinary vessels. In modern Chinese tradition there is less specific reference to this distinct separation of root and local treatments in practice. Obviously, the concept is present and used. The open point systems that are still in use in China and the diagnoses of underlying dysfunctions that give rise to symptoms are both evidences of this concept. Dr. Zhang Xin Shu, who has developed a treatment system where six pairs of points on the arms and legs are treated to control various body zones, describes these points as root treatment points. His book *Wan Ke Zhen, Wrist Ankle Acupuncture*, will be discussed later.

Although related by the idea of root treatments, element or meridian problems are not equivalent to extraordinary vessel disease. The *Nan Jing* was first to state this distinction clearly. The meridian system and the diagnostic and therapeutic theories of the five elements represent a different energetic strata than the extraordinary vessels. Though all the energetic systems share an origin in the center, problems that manifest in the branch systems are not necessarily problems of the center:

> *If the {twelve} meridians are full, {replete, overflowing}, this fullness {spills over} goes into the eight extraordinary vessels, never to return.*[26]

In the *Nan Jing* the extraordinary vessels were believed to function like the system of dikes that was used in China to drain fields when rivers overflowed. The yin and yang qiao mai, which were seen as two of the fifteen luo vessels described in the *Nan Jing*,[27] were particularly important, being the first to receive the energy that spilled over.[28] However, later discussions make little note of this function.

This was the earliest attempt to rationalize a general function for the extraordinary vessels. Earlier discussions had focussed on the individual functions of the extraordinary vessels. The *Nan Jing* attempted to place these vessels in the context of a global view of the human body.

This idea may be represented by a series of diagrams. The tai yi, the great one, starts to separate at the level of no-form. It then divides to become the two, yin and yang. Yin and yang then divide twice. On the one hand, the two become the three, the three warmers, their associated qi and functions. The three divide to become the six, the five elements and their source, or the six pairs of meridians: tai yang, shao yang, yang ming, tai yin, shao yin, and jue yin. These pairs further divide producing the twelve meridians. On the other hand, the second branch of the yin—yang division becomes the four, the divisions of the body, which become the eight, the extraordinary vessels.

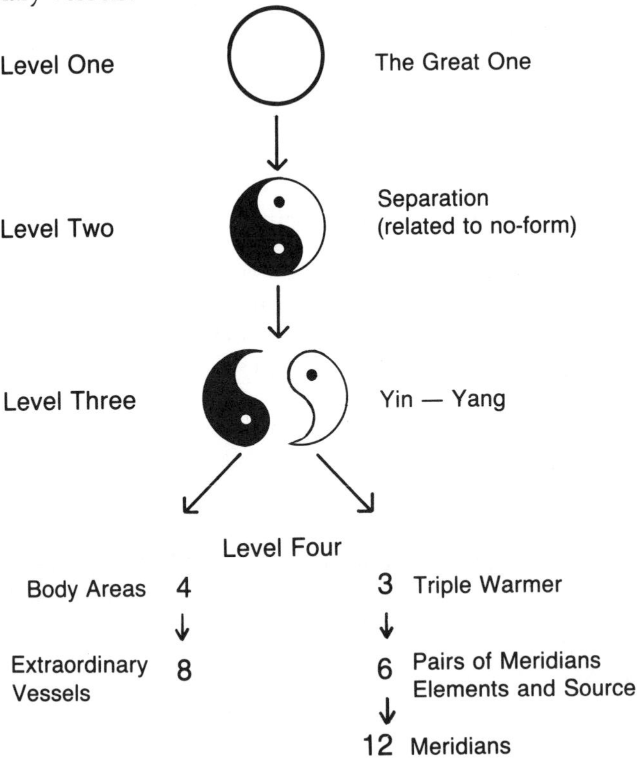

Figure 3

Using any of these pathways we can treat the root. The means chosen depends on the specific imbalance. Local treatments are somewhat outside of this scheme. However, clinical experience indicates that local treatments work much better if the root problem is corrected first, or simultaneously. Modern treatments provide two basic approaches for reaching root problems through the extraordinary vessels. The first style we have chosen to represent this methodology is the work of Ms. Michi Tokito. She works at the level of no-form, before the first division of yin—yang, water—fire. Imbalances determined by the five element theory are treated simultaneously with the extraordinary vessels. The second style, represented by the work of Mr. Osamu Ito, includes the use of extraordinary vessel treatments supplemented by adjunctive local treatment. To this system we have added a methodology for simultaneous five element treatment. Though simple, these treatment procedures have profound effects. Each system is based in the essential understanding of the *Nan Jing*: all energies begin in the center.

The Extraordinary Vessels and Body Structure

It is not absolutely possible to distinguish the energetic structure of the body from the material structure. Practitioners have noticed that treating the extraordinary vessels frequently corrects structural problems such as tension, right—left imbalance, length differences or postural quirks. This discovery is both recent and intriguing. Using ion cords on the extraordinary vessels will release muscle tension in areas that had been tense on palpation. Using electrically active metals and magnets on the extraordinary vessels ameliorates imbalances of the neck, lower back and knees. The patient's physical bearing adjusts as these treatments relieve structural stress. These experiences directed attention to various classical discussions of the structure of the extraordinary vessels, yielding through research both a better understanding and a therapeutic advance.

Dr. Manaka developed this understanding of the extraordinary meridians from a topological approach. If we look at the eight extraordinary vessel pathways, we become quickly aware of a certain symmetry. There is a vessel that ascends the front of the body on the midline – the ren mai. One ascends the back on the midline – the du mai. A horizontal vessel circles the body around the waist – the dai mai. Thus may we derive a basic picture of the body:

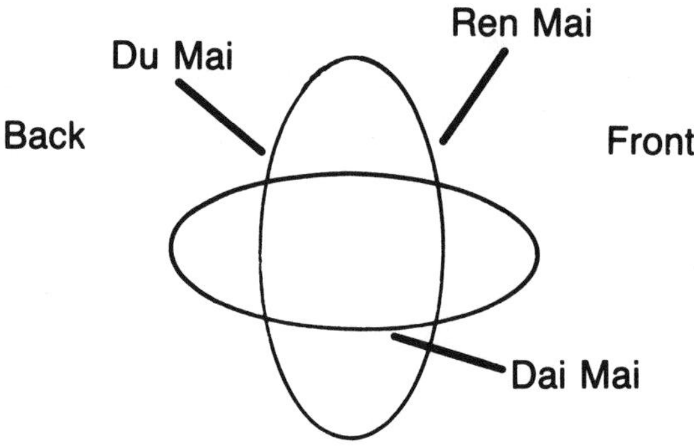

Figure 4

In further development of this idea, Dr. Manaka discusses these divisions in relation to the right and left sides of the body, the upper and lower, front and back.[29] He maps the body in eight sections or areas, coining the term "octants."

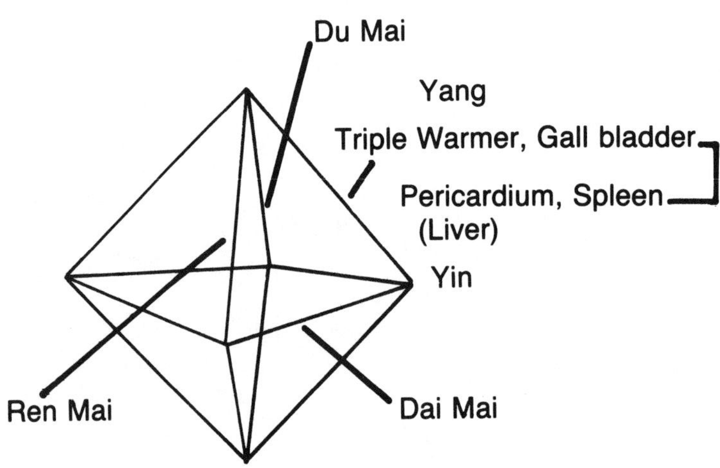

Figure 5

The eight extraordinary vessels directly relate to these eight areas of the body. In effect, the ren and du mai divide the left and right sides of the body. The dai mai divides the upper and lower parts of the body. The gallbladder and triple warmer meridians divide the front and back parts of the yang aspect. The pericardium and liver meridians divide the front and back parts of the yin aspect.[30] The treatment points of the yin and yang wei mai lie on the pericardium and triple warmer meridians, PC-6 and TW-5 respectively. The treatment points of the chong mai and the dai mai are found on the spleen and gall bladder meridians, SP-4 and GB-41. This parallels the idea that these four meridians divide the front and back portions of the yin and yang aspects of the body. The sole exception is SP-4. Theoretically, the liver meridian would be a better fit. However, the spleen meridian has a similar pathway up the inside of the legs and travels higher and closer to the energetic center as it ascends the trunk. Thus, these four extraordinary vessels divide the front and back sides of the body and connect the upper and lower parts. The yin and yang qiao mai, through their connections to the kidney and bladder meridians (their treatment points are KI-6 and BL-62) have strong relationships to the ren and du mai. The trajectory of the kidney meridian is proximate to the ren mai. The bladder meridian is equally close to the du mai.[31] Thus, these too relate to the front and back, upper and lower portions of the body.

Understanding this connection has important consequences in treatment, as this knowledge helps to differentiate problems of the eight extraordinary vessels from problems of the twelve meridians. When thinking of the twelve meridians and the five yin and six yang organs, we are thinking in terms of corresponding functions and symptoms. When thinking about the extraordinary vessels we are advised to relate the eight extraordinary vessels to the eight areas of the body. This appropriately implies that there is a greater physical element to the function of the extraordinary vessels. Since the extraordinary vessels are at a deeper level in the energetic strata of the human body, they are more closely allied to the formative energies; their function is broader and strongly related to the growth of the physical form. Many practitioners who have become expert at the use of the extraordinary vessels have relied on palpation, for it is this method of assessment that most directly accesses information about balance and form.

Thus, to diagnose the extraordinary meridians, we should focus our attention on body balance and symmetry. When we treat the extraordinary vessels we restore balance. In the differentiation process, we should not inordinately attend to the nature of the person's disease, but concern ourselves with the patient's bodily imbalances. Let us remark here that Dr. Manaka is the first to note this approach is an heuristic methodology, not an immobile truth. We can affect energetics and body balance by treating either meridians and organs or areas and octants. However, since this principle is useful in practice and often provides the desired results, it is a good starting point for therapeutic problem solving.[32]

In our problem solving we may not forget that at least three of the extraordinary vessels have a direct relationships to the twelve meridians. The du mai is the ocean of the yang; the ren mai is the ocean of the yin; the chong mai is the ocean of the twelve meridians, the five yin and six yang organs, the ocean of blood, and the moving qi between the kidneys. These relationships were discussed by Li Shi Zhen, who saw the ren, du and chong mai as interrelated:

> *The triple warmer is the function of ming men. The ren mai and du mai make contact together at the chong mai.*[33]

He explains this statement by noting that the ren mai and du mai are the fundamental divisions of yin and yang in the body. The chong mai insures the inseparability or oneness of the ren and du mai, the yin and yang functions:

> *The ren mai and du mai are the "midday and midnight" (wu [午] and zi [子]) of the body. The ren mai and du mai are the polar axis of the body. Mr. Hua says, "The ren and du mai are two vessels. {There is} one source, consequently two branches. One movement goes to the front of the body, one movement goes to the back of the body. The body has the ren and du mai just as heaven and earth have the midday and midnight. Using these we can divide the body, day and night. We can also make connections between them. When we try to divide these, we see that yin and yang are inseparable. When we try to see them as one, we see that it is an indivisible whole. This is why there is one and consequently two, two and consequently one."*[34]

Again, the ren and du mai represent the basic division of yin and yang in the body. They stem from a single source, the moving qi between the kidneys, the chong mai. This helps us understand the *Su Wen* discussion of the branch of the "main vessel" of the du mai that follows the ren mai trajectory; yin and yang are inseparable.[35] Ultimately, both are the same and have the same source; they represent the yin and yang components of the same vessel. This also helps us understand Wang Bing's commentary on the *Su Wen*:

> *This is why we can say the du mai, ren mai and chong mai have different names but are all the same.*[36]

This is really a statement about their common origin in the abdomen at the moving qi between the kidneys, the uterus. In effect, the classical authors were describing a central energetic field that was named and differentiated by function.

Li Shi Zhen's ideas about the extraordinary vessels differ slightly from those presented in the *Zhen Jiu Da Quan*. He did not use the eight treatment points, nor did he use the ling gui ba fa (eight methods of the spiritual turtle) biorhythmic treatments; he treated principally with internal medicine. However, his theoretical understanding fits well with the general theory.

Modern topological ideas merge the *Da Quan* and Li Shi Zhen with modern practice. They allow us to see the inseparability of the body's structure and energy. This synthesis is particularly clear when we examine the extraordinary vessels from a developmental perspective. The progressive physical development of the human embryo occurs in stages that also describe the energetic development. The inseparability of structure and energy is clear.

The first division of the fertilized ovum produces the ren and du mai, the second the dai mai.[37] The work of Tohaku Ishi and others shows a probable relationship of the ren and du mai to the primordial tissues of early development, tracing the connections of the ren and du mai to the anterior and posterior hypophysis and thus the endocrine system.[38] These relationships are natural extensions of the topological conception of the extraordinary vessels. The form and structure of the body begin and mature together.

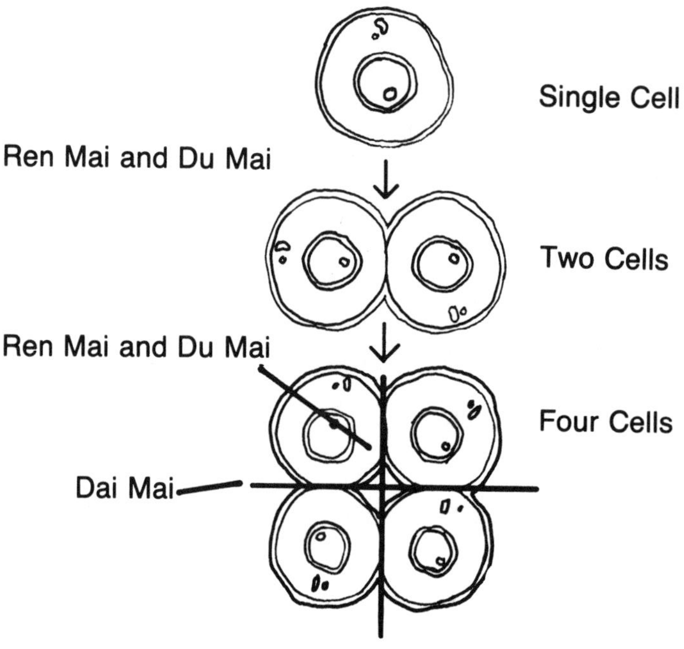

Figure 6

While the technology to demonstrate bioelectrical activity in the first cells of animal life is available and has shown such activity, ethical considerations bar research into the bioelectrical activity of the first cells of human life. Thus, data is not available to prove this idea. However, clinical practice demonstrates that treatments based on this assumption are effective. Regardless of the availability of material evidence, clearly the structural aspects of the extraordinary vessels indicate that there are extremely subtle and pervasive forces at work. In addition, the association of extraordinary vessel development with prenatal and conceptional energies helps to explain the relationship of these vessels to biorhythmic patterns as well as the emphasis on prenatal, cosmological energies that is found in the classical texts.

Extraordinary Vessel Biorhythms

The theory of biorhythmic influences is well known. These rhythms are thought to be established by complex external cycles — the rotation of the earth, the rotation of the moon around the earth, the rotation of both around the sun and the progression of the sun along the celestial equator. These cycles are incorporated into the Chinese calendar, into astronomical science and into the stem and branch systems in medicine. In Eastern thought the concepts of qi, rhythmicity and energetic environment provide the rationale for the biorhythmic effects noted. In Western thought, esoteric ideas such as "rays" or "influences" provide the explanatory mechanism in occult systems. The concept of fields is the explanation of science.

The principal factor common to these cycles is the geomagnetic field of the earth. Considerable research has shown how the body is sensitive to variations in the geomagnetic field; many biological functions are conditioned by geomagnetic fluctuations. It is reasonable to suppose that the physical body may be affected by these field variations through the energetic system. Biorhythms would be thus the cyclic response to changes in the geomagnetic field; particularly, the biorhythmic fluctuations of the meridian and extraordinary vessel systems.[39] By understanding the biorhythms of Chinese medical theory, we may better understand the meridians and extraordinary vessels.

The body's tai yi, the moving qi, is a reflection of the tai yi of Chinese astronomy, a microcosmic reflection of the macrocosm. The mechanism of this reflection is the ability of one energy to affect another, particularly in the closely allied system of heaven—person—earth. Both Xu Feng's biorhythmic system and Dr. Manaka's topological theory may be explained through the *Nan Jing* idea of a central source and its ability to respond to external energies. If we conceive of this source as an ocean, or in more modern terms an energetic field, we may posit that it is capable of responding to both internal and external influences. The idea of a heaven—person—earth triad implies that the meeting of heavenly and earthly influences in the person is mutually interactive. The source receives and transmits signals. Small biases and minor gradients, even perhaps those as small as the early bioelectrical patterns of the ovum, result in the channelling of the body's energies in predictable patterns.

As the *Nan Jing* describes, each of the meridian and organ systems branches through the body from this source. Just as the patterns of heavenly influence were described as stems and branches, the patterns of energetic influence in the human body are the stems and branches of the source. Through these the function of the whole may be affected. The extraordinary vessels are a specific aspect of this complex and subtle interchange of signals.

Here, the idea of a field is of considerable use. While field descriptions and theories are often mathematical and complex, the idea itself is simple. A field is an area where an energy or energies are active, or potentially active. There are many well known examples. The field of a magnet and the gravitational field of the earth are both generally known. Less understood, and more recently discovered, are the fields that surround biological life. In the human body, the heart, brain, muscles and the retina of the eye each produce a field that may be measured outside the body with sensitive magnetometers. In effect, a field is a space where energies or objects that enter the area are acted upon in some way. The action that occurs varies according to the type of field, energy or object that interacts. In every instance, the field is a description of the force that is exerted upon the energy or object influenced.

In the present context, we may conceive of the human energetic system as a complex field, thus creating a picture of the relationships and interactions theorized in acupuncture. The heaven— person— earth triad may be seen as a diagram of potential interaction between three fields. The mutuality of the interaction is the result of their association; a change or stimulus in one field will affect the "overlapping" fields. Some of these stimuli will be energetic, that is, the quantity or quality of the energies will be changed. For example, absorbing or diminishing the quantity of an energy in one part of the field will have an effect not only on the other parts of that field, but also on any other field the interaction of which is in some way dependent on the quantity of the diminished energy. In many ways the self regulating nature of the five element phases is a description of a field where various deficits or excesses change the distribution of energy in the field.

Other interactions will be informational. For example, if the metabolism of an organism is in some way determined by the temperature of the surrounding atmosphere, cooling that atmosphere will not diminish the energy, the amount of the signal, but the organism's response will change. The idea of "cold invasion" comes to mind easily. While the external perverse cold energy does enter the meridian, that is, a material change of the meridian energy occurs, there are also changes in the function of other elements of the meridian system that are not directly invaded. The existence of the cold in the meridian signals defensive adaptations. In this regard the classical idea of defense or wei qi clearly has a warning or informational function.

The *Nan Jing* and subsequent descriptions of human energetic interrelations are easily conceived as overlapping fields. The level of no-form is entirely energetic and informational, the exchange between microcosm and macrocosm is most powerfully organizational. The division of yin and yang, fire and water, is also predominantly an exchange of information, the quality of the result is determined by the relative mix of the potentials described by these symbols. Ming men, the hara, the uterus, the oceans of qi and blood represent a more material, yet still predominantly energetic set of relationships and exchanges. These are the fields within the field of no-form. In turn, the triple warmer, master of the heart and the eight extraordinary vessels have a dual role. In some instances we are concerned with the quality and quantity of the energy, in other instances we are concerned with their role as an information network. If the triple warmer energy carried to the source points is excess or deficient, the resulting imbalance will be material, or metabolic. If the energy is sufficient, yet mistimed or misdirected, the result will be the malfunction of the systems that depend on its signals for their function.

In the extraordinary vessels, some of the ascribed functions are metabolic, the interchange of energy. Others are informational. In their role as "seas" they effect the distribution of qi. As topological entities they provide for the exchange of information throughout the organism. As with all Chinese energetic concepts these two functions are neither completely distinct nor separable. One salient point of the classical theorists is that such a separation is more conceptual than real. However, by understanding the extraordinary vessels as fields within fields that are capable of both changing the distribution and quality of energy used in the body and changing the signals that control the use of that energy, we are able to understand the broadest range of therapeutic options. To take advantage of this realization, we must become familiar with the extraordinary vessel pathways.

Notes

[1] The master points were first described in the *Zhen Jiu Da Quan,* 1439 AD.

[2] Li Shi Zhen, *Qi Jing Ba Mai Kao.* See *Pulse Diagnosis* for Li Shi Zhen's pulse diagnosis of the extraordinary vessels.

[3] This subsequent text, *Hara, Reflections on the Sea* is due for publication in 1986.

[4] Our brief study is based on studies found in the *Morohashi Encyclopedic Dictionary, Fujido's Etymological Dictionary* and the *Kadokawa Etymological Dictionary.*

[5] See for instance, *Su Wen* Chapters 44, 60 and *Ling Shu* Chapters 2, 10, 11, 17, 21, 33, 38, 62, 65.

[6] Wang Shu He, *Mai Jing,* vol. 2, pp. 15-16.

[7] Li Shi Zhen, *Qi Jing Ba Mai Kao,* p. 27.

[8] Henri Maspero supports this relationship. See *Taoism and Chinese Religion.*

[9] Wang Shu He, *Commentary on Nan Jing,* Chapters 28 and 29.

[10] The style, called the *ling gui ba fa,* the "eight methods of the spiritual turtle." was also found in the later *Da Cheng* text.

[11] Wang Shu He presents what is probably the first idea of extraordinary vessel biorhythms. *Commentary on Nan Jing,* Chapter 27, vol. 2, p. 13 *passim.*

[12] *Zhen Jiu Da Quan,* pp. 128-129.

[13] *Ibid.,* pp. 131-132.

[14] *Ibid.*

[15] *Zhen Jiu Da Cheng,* p. 43, derived from the earlier text, the *Zhen Jing Zhi Nan,* p. 146.

[16] *Zhen Jing Zhi Nan,* pp. 155-165. Found in the *Zhen Jiu Si Shu,* the *Four Books of Acupuncture and Moxibustion* compiled by Dou Jie before 1311 AD. Much of the discussion from the *Zhen Jing Zhi Nan*

seems to have been absorbed by the *Zhen Jiu Ju Ying* of 1529. It also influenced the *Zhen Jiu Da Cheng.* The term Zhi Nan, "South Pointer" refers to a compass. See J. Needham; *Science and Civilization in China*, vol. IV, part 1, pp. 269-271.

[17] *Nan Jing,* Chapter 8 *passim.*

[18] *Ibid.,*, Chapters 25 and 38.

[19] *Zhuang Zi,* Chapter 17, p. 378, quoted from *Lao Zi, Zhuang Zi,* p. 378.

[20] *Huai Nan Zi,* Chapter 2, p. 59, with Haruki Kusuyama's commentary.

[21] *Ibid.*, p. 61.

[22] *Lie Zi,* "Tian Shui" chapter, cited from the *Morohashi Encyclopedic Dictionary.*

[23] *Huai Nan Zi,*, Chapter 7, p. 338.

[24] See Bohm, *Wholeness and the Implicate Order,* and Wilber, ed., *Holographic Paradigm and Other Paradoxes.*

[25] *Su Wen,* Chapter 5, p. 32.

[26] *Nan Jing,* Chapter 28, vol. 2, p. 16.

[27] *Ibid.*, Chapter 27.

[28] *Ibid.*, See also, Wang Shu He, *Commentary on Nan Jing.*

[29] Yoshio Manaka, MD, PhD, *Ika no Tameno Shinjutsu Nyumon Kuoza,* pp. 14-15.

[30] *Ibid.,* p. 356. Although these relationships are obvious when presented to us, they were not systematically stated or implied in any therapeutic style until the Ming Dynasty. The *Zhen Jiu Da Quan, The Complete text of Acupuncture and Moxibustion,* first discussed this relationship in the context of the eight master points that we commonly use to treat problems associated with the extraordinary vessels.

[31] *Ibid.*, p. 358.

[32] *Ibid.*, p. 14-15.

[33] Li Shi Zhen, *Qi Jing Ba Mai Kao,*, vol. 1, p. 14.

[34] *Ibid.*, vol. 1, p. 21. Mr. Hua is the author of the *Shisi Jing Fa Hui*

[35] *Su Wen,* Chapter 60 *passim* and Wang Bing's *Commentary.*

[36] Wang Bing, quoted from the *Nei Jing Jie Po Sheng Li Xue,* p. 121.

[37] Y. Manaka MD, PhD, "Shinkyu kenkyu ni oyoshita jiki kotoni sono keiketsu sessyoku koka ni tsuite" (pamphlet handed out at his lectures).

[38] Y. Manaka, MD, PhD, *Shinkyu no riron to kangaikata,* p. 68.

[39] In *Hara, Reflections on the Sea,* biorhythms are discussed as correlations between the classical Chinese concepts of stems and branches and modern notions of geomagnetic and other fields. A very good summary of geomagnetic field effects can be found in A. P. Dubrov, *The Geomagnetic Field and Life: Geomagnetobiology*, New York, Plenum Press, 1978.

Extraordinary Vessel Trajectories

Concerning the internal and external paths of the twelve meridians, consensus points to the accuracy of the information in the *Ling Shu* and the *Shisi Jing Fa Hui, Elucidation of the Fourteen Meridians* of 1341 AD. Concerning the extraordinary vessels, there has never been such a precise consensus. Since there have been many interpretations of the earliest explanations of the extraordinary vessels from the *Su Wen, Ling Shu* and *Nan Jing,* determining their trajectories is not an easy undertaking. Nonetheless, the main sources for this information must be the earlier classics. As additional sources, we have a preference for Wang Shu He's *Commentary on the Nan Jing* and Li Shi Zhen's text on the eight extraordinary vessels, the *Qi Jing Ba Mai Kao.* We have also used the *Lei Jing,* or *Classic of Categories.* The modern Chinese text, *Nei Jing Jie Po Sheng Li Xue, Anatomy and Physiology of the Su Wen,* has a good compilation of the major sources and commentaries.

It is important to remember that all these great texts are the written record of the experience and observation of their authors. Thus, in addition to the problems of translating a character language, where there is no absolute certainty that the modern meaning of a character is indeed its ancient meaning, there are the problems inherent in any language. Describing the energetic pathways of the human body in words, or in two dimensional drawings, is no simple task. The mental exercise required to reduce a three dimensional form to words or artistic representation is subject to considerable uncertainty. Is a line on the side of the face behind the lips on the front of the face, or is it at the front of the side? Though a practitioner or author may easily recognize or locate the indications of a pathway, often he cannot precisely describe this knowledge in a chart or expression.

This is further complicated by the pathway or meridian concept itself. When we write or teach, we find the idea of a channel to be useful. Yet, are there really channels? Are we discussing some physical analog of the meridian concept, if so, is this analog an actual, linear path that contains the energy flow as an aquaduct contains water? Since what we expect to "flow in the meridians" is an energy, an extremely subtle energy, such a physical conduit is unlikely. Further, physical channels have not been found. What has been found is different electrical properties in areas that correspond to the Oriental medical concepts of points and meridians.[1] If we are to discuss the flow of energy and ascribe lateral and vertical direction to it, to allocate points along its path and posit the results of stimulating those points, we need to propose some idea of how this energy moves.

We begin with the presumption that when we are discussing meridians we are discussing gradients. Further, these gradients operate within fields, areas of potential influence. Qi, while it may be much more than electricity, is similar to electricity in that it can be described as moving from an area of greater or lesser potential to an area of a complementary and opposite potential. This is simply another yin—yang pair. Thus, meridians may be thought of as the path of least resistance between gradients. Depending on the source and polarity, energy passes from yin to yang, yang to yin, and the meridian is the resulting course. The meridian description as a line or channel is a practical means of describing and organizing the phenomena by which we observe the transference of this energy.

This is particularly true of the extraordinary vessels. Often they are described as seas or oceans, clearly implying that the energy is at least more broadly channeled. Their intimate connection to the tai yi and their strong relationship to biorhythmic influences also suggest fields and gradients more strongly than absolute channels. The classical disagreements among commentators who have described the extraordinary vessels should not be taken as an issue of who is right or wrong. First, some allowance must be made for the linguistic problem of reporting a phenomenon that was largely inferred, rather than anatomically traced. Second, we must not allow the words of our organizing concept, "meridian," "channel," or "vessel," to misrepresent the phenomena by implying too strongly a physically fixed or absolute line. The line we use to draw the picture is not the meridian. In this sense, "vessel," which implies a larger, less linear container, is a better choice of word. Finally, we must also consider that these vessels are two dimensional only when we describe them in words or drawings. In operation, they are three dimensional and may be wider or thinner at various places along their trajectories.

In response to local gradients, variations in potential, a meridian could be less a channel and more an area. Thus, these energetic seas and oceans may have their own topography, now a stream, now a river and later perhaps a broad sea. It is useful to remember the concept of a field when thinking of meridians. As noted earlier, this idea from energetic physics is three dimensional and represents an area of kinetic or potential energy. While fields are often found in relation to material forms and structures, they are entirely energetic.

They are shaped by the energetic potentials that are their source and are able to influence other fields. Thus, the idea of a field satisfies all the criteria of a meridian in classical medical thought and provides the conceptual tools necessary to consider energy flow without the limits inherent in the word "channel." If we keep in mind the idea of a field when discussing meridian trajectories, we are able to understand that frequently all the variant opinions regarding a meridian path may be no more than different, partial descriptions of the same phenomenon.

Ren Mai

The *Su Wen* tells us this about the ren mai, or "conception vessel," as it is known in English:

> *The ren mai starts below zhongji {CV-3}. It then comes up from the edge of the hair {the superior edge of the pubic hairs on the midline}, circles along the lining of the abdomen and comes up to guanyuan {CV-4}. Then it passes up to the throat, circles around the chin, then around the face, and enters the eyes.*[2]

There are a variety of ideas concerning the origin of the ren mai. The *Ling Shu* tells us that it originates from the uterus;[3] at least, this is how most readers understand the *Lei Jing* interpretation of the expression, "The chong mai and ren mai start at the covering of the small abdomen."[4] Other interpreters feel that this vessel begins above GV-1.[5] The writer of the *Tai Su* says, "Below the zhongji, this is the inside of the womb."[6] Li Shi Zhen, who described the most detailed trajectory for the vessel, felt that "below zhongji" was too vague, and that the ren mai began at CV-1,[7] and that it became the ocean or controller of the yin meridians:[8]

> *{It occurs} below zhongji (inside the small abdomen) which is the dividing place of huiyin {CV-1}. It rises up and comes to the surface of the abdomen at qugu {CV-2}, up the edge of the hair to zhongji, rising superficially through the lining of the abdomen, circling outwards to the spleen, kidney and liver meridians. Then to guanyuan; then to shimen {CV-5}. Shimen is dantian, one more name for it is ming men. It is two divisions below the umbilicus and is a mu point of the triple*

> *warmer. Then up to qihai {CV-6}; to yinjiao {CV-7}, meeting with the gallbladder meridian and the chong mai, which is also the entrance of the bladder and a mu point of the triple warmer. Then it rises up to shenque {CV-8}, to shuifen, to xiawan {CV-10}, where it meets the spleen meridian; then up to jianli, to zhongwan {CV-12}, meeting the lung, triple warmer and stomach meridians; then to shangwan {CV-13}, up through the points to tiantu {CV-22} and lianquan {CV-23}, where it meets the yin wei mai. Then it travels up the chin to chengjiang {CV-24}, meeting with the du mai, large intestine and stomach meridians; then it circles around the lips on the inside of the mouth, divides and passes up to chengqi {ST-1} where it ends.*[9]

The *Nan Jing* trajectory description, which is based on an expansion of ideas from Chapter 60 of the *Su Wen*, varies slightly from Li Shi Zhen's description. Instead of dividing around the inside of the mouth, as is proposed by Li Shi Zhen, the *Nan Jing* states that the ren mai comes up the throat and chin, then splits and rises to enter the eyes. From here it branches to circulate through the tongue.[10]

Another important variation of the trajectory comes from the *Ling Shu*:

> *The tail shadow {dividing luo meridian} of the ren mai goes to pigeon tail {CV-15} and from there goes into the abdomen. . . For excess conditions, the abdominal skin will be painful; for deficient conditions, there will be itching.*[11]

Ren Mai Points		
Trajectory	**Point**	**Source**
Starts	CV-1	*Qi Jing Ba Mai Kao*
	ST-30	Wang Shu He
Passes through	CV-1 to CV-24	Most sources
Ends	ST-1	*Qi Jing Ba Mai Kao*
Luo point	CV-15	*Ling Shu*

There are a some important questions regarding the association of the ren mai with ST-30. These are discussed in the next section.

Ren Mai Trajectory

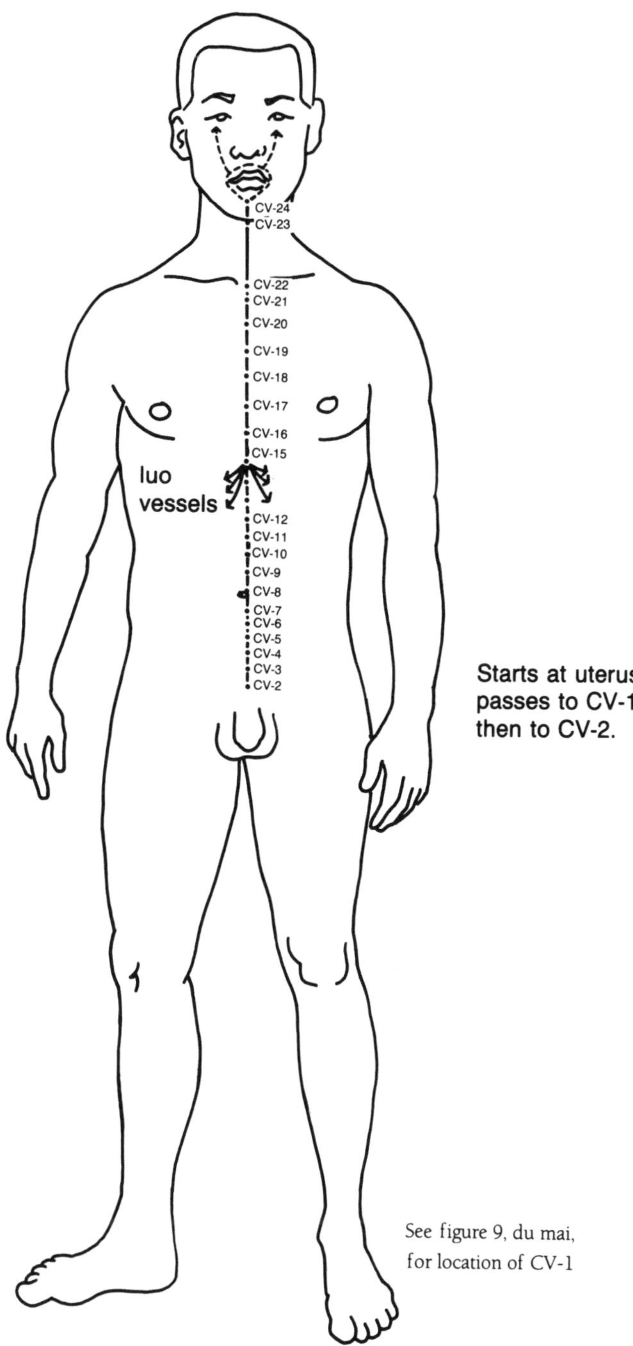

See figure 9, du mai, for location of CV-1

Figure 7

The Chong Mai

We read in the *Su Wen*:

> *The chong mai begins at qichong {ST-30}, comes up, on, or close to the kidney meridian on either side of the umbilicus, reaches to and goes into the chest, then disperses.*[12]

Different interpretations and alternate trajectories exist. The *Ling Shu* defines the chong mai and details a trajectory:

> *The chong mai is the ocean of the five yin organs and six yang organs, the ocean of the twelve meridians, and passes blood to the five yin and six yang organs. It rises up the neck and chin, moistens each of the yang {meridians} and moistens each of the jing. Then a branch passes down, this is the big luo of shao yin, and comes out at qichong (ST-30). A branch goes down inside the thigh, entering behind the knee, going down through the liver bone of the leg, to the internal malleolus. Then it separates. One branch runs alongside the kidney meridian, moistening the three yin. The other branch comes to the upper surface of the foot and then goes down into the foot between the first and second toes.*[13]

It is unclear whether "the big luo of shao yin" is related to the heart or the kidney meridian, a factor which will feature in following discussions. The author of the *Lei Jing* comments that the "three yin" moistened by the chong mai are the three yin meridians of the leg.[14]

The *Ling Shu* presents a similar but abbreviated description:

> *The chong mai is the ocean of the twelve meridians and the big luo of the shao yin. It comes from below the kidneys and rises to the surface at ST-30; then passes down inside the thigh to behind the knee, down inside the tibia to behind the internal malleolus, where it divides. One branch goes down the kidney meridian, the other to the upper surface of the foot and down between the first and second toes, keeping the lower leg warm.*[15]

There is another passage from the *Ling Shu* concerning the trajectory of the chong mai, which is perhaps more difficult to understand because of the one-sided pathway description:

> *The chong mai and ren mai originate from the inside of the uterus, a branch rises up in front of the spine making the "ocean of the twelve meridians." The branch that floats up to the surface of the abdomen only rises up the right side and then reunites {with the ren mai} at the throat; then it separates and circles around the lips.*[16]

Finally, in the "Four Ocean" chapter of the *Ling Shu*, the chong mai is again described as the "ocean of the twelve meridians" and the "ocean of blood." Upper and lower "shu" or transportation points are also described. These could be either treatment or pathway points, the passage is not totally clear:

> *The chong mai is the ocean of the twelve meridians, its upper {transportation} shu point is dashu {BL-11}, and its lower shu points are shangjuxu {ST-37} and tiaokou {ST-38}. . .*
>
> *{In a condition of} excess blood, the body feels full; {in a condition of} deficient blood, the body feels small.*[17]

These passages from the *Su Wen* and *Ling Shu* have been accepted in large part; however, they have been interpreted and further elaborated in a variety of ways. Some commentators disagree with others. The *Nan Jing* says only that:

> *The chong mai starts at qijie [氣街], {which many see as ST-30} and rises parallel to the stomach meridian, surrounds the umbilicus, then goes inside the chest to disperse.*[18]

This terse statement by the *Nan Jing* is expanded slightly by Wang Shu He in his *Commentary on the Nan Jing*:

> *The du mai, ren mai and chong mai start at qijie. This point is the three branching point of the source.*[19]

He also comments, "Chong mai is the general of the twelve meridians."[20] This indicates that he thought of the chong mai as governing all the meridians in some fashion. He expresses this concept more clearly in his *Mai Jing, Classic of the Pulse.* There, he sees the joint function of the du and chong mai as essential to the circulation of the twelve meridians:

> *The chong and du mai combined are the "way" of the twelve meridians. If the chong and du mai do not function correctly, the twelve meridians do not return to the great meeting of the vessels (LU-9).*[21]

Relative to the chong mai trajectory, qijie is seen as another name for ST-30, which is usually called qichong [氣衝]. The character chong in qichong is the same as the character chong of chong mai. The character jie has some interesting meanings. It is generally seen to mean a thoroughfare, a wide or large street.[22] Etymologically, it is derived from the idea of a crossroads.[23] Thus, qijie implies a qi crossroad or thoroughfare. This is further emphasized by the idea of "street" or "passing" attached to the character chong. To understand this concept fully we should examine the *Ling Shu* discussion of the several jie in the body:

> *To explain about qijie: in the chest the qi has a jie; in the abdomen the qi has a jie; in the head the qi has a jie; in the lower part of the legs the qi has a jie. Therefore, qi is in the head. {If there is a problem of} qi in the head, stop this at the brain.*
>
> *{If there is a problem of} qi in the chest, stop this at the front of the chest and at the back-shu points.*
>
> *{If there is a problem of} qi in the abdomen, stop this at the back shu points and at the moving vessel at the right and left sides of the umbilicus, the chong mai.*
>
> *{If there is a problem of} qi in the lower parts of the legs, stop this at qijie {possibly ST-30} and at chengshan {BL-57}, and above or below the malleoli. Treat these by inserted needle techniques. Before one inserts, rub {the point} for a long time; then when one's hand feels something, insert the needle.*[24]

Some commentators feel that "stop this at the brain" means to treat GV-20. We feel that it refers to GV-17 and, or GB-19, "brain door" and "brain emptiness." The same passage goes on to give some symptoms of qijie: headache, dizziness, abdominal pain, fullness in the abdomen, severe swelling.[25] Thus, qijie seems to be a meeting place of qi. The various locations of the qijie in the body, the head, chest, abdomen and lower legs, imply some process of condensation or meeting of the qi in those areas. The condensation or collection of qi causes the symptoms mentioned.

After studying this passage, it is hard to accept qijie as ST-30. Qijie seems to be more a concept of collection of qi. What these places are and what their functions may be is hard to determine. Little is generally said about qijie, except that it is ST-30. Perhaps various commentators see it as ST-30 because of the quotes from the *Su Wen* and the *Ling Shu* that state the relationship of the chong mai to ST-30, qichong. But we are not convinced that this is exactly what the *Nan Jing* and Wang Shu He had in mind. It would probably be more useful to see ST-30 not as the starting place of the chong mai, but as the first acupoint on its pathway, as the passages from the *Ling Shu* seem to imply.

That the du mai, ren mai and chong mai all start at qijie is also hard to interpret. Li Shi Zhen as well as Gao Wu, the author of the *Zhen Jiu Ju Ying, Gathering of Eminent Acupuncturists,* feel that the chong mai starts at CV-1.[26] However, the *Ling Shu* states that the chong mai starts at the area "below the kidneys"[27] and from the "inside of the womb."[28] Considering all these interpretations we can see qijie as being inside the body, below the kidneys, or at the inside of the womb, an understanding offered by the *Tai Su*. This text posits the chong mai as originating inside the womb, thus beginning from the source, the moving qi between the kidneys — the central focus of the energetic body, the root of life and movement.[29] If we accept this idea, we can make sense of Wang Shu He's comment that the du mai, ren mai and chong mai all start at qijie. Each would thus begin at the uterus, the moving qi between the kidneys.

This becomes more complicated when we look at other discussions of the qijie as seen relative to the zong qi and its movement through the body:

> *The zong qi collects at the ocean {upper qihai}. The zong qi that goes to the lower parts goes to qijie. The zong qi that goes to the upper parts runs into the throat. Therefore, if there is rebellious, obstructed qi in the leg, the zong qi does not pass downwards, the blood in the vessels becomes stuck and stops moving. Only by using fire {moxa} can you control {this}.*[30]

If we see qijie as ST-30, then ST-30 must also be a meeting point for the zong qi. If, as we suggest, qijie is an energetic center in the body, the moving qi between the kidneys, the idea of collection of qi makes more sense. We cannot ignore that most commentators say qijie is ST-30. Perhaps ST-30 is a reflex point for the qijie; it is at least a treatment point for the lower leg jie.

The abdominal pathway of the chong mai that ascends to the chest, the face, and down the legs is also of some interest. Neither the *Nan Jing* nor Wang Shu He comment on the trajectory of the chong mai up the abdomen. We can only assume that the earlier descriptions were accepted and required no comment. This is not true for later commentaries. The *Zhen Jiu Jia Yi Jing*, the *Systematic Classic of Acupuncture and Moxibustion*, compiled circa 282 AD, disagrees with the *Ling Shu* idea that it only rises up the right side of the abdomen.[31] This text indicates that it rises along both sides of the abdomen, as the *Su Wen* says. Li Shi Zhen also supported this concept.[32] The *Lei Jing* adopts the *Ling Shu* idea with an interesting comment:

> *The chong mai and ren mai are yin, yang (complements), therefore the chong mai comes up the right side of the abdomen and the big luo of the stomach goes to the left side, below the breast. {This} is left-yang, right-yin, this is the balance of the body.*[33]

An important concept is contained in this idea. Left-yang, right-yin is a theory that comes to us from Chapter Five, the "Great Phenomena of Yin and Yang" chapter of the *Su Wen*. The idea of the "big luo of the stomach" also comes from the *Su Wen*:

> *The big luo of the stomach is called xu li [虛里] {empty li, mile}. It passes through the diaphragm and spirally wraps the lungs. Then it comes out below the left breast.*[34]

This passage continues, describing the pulsing or palpitation that can be seen or felt at this place. Because of this association some researchers feel that the big luo of the stomach is the pacemaker of the heart. If the pulsing is too large, particularly if it is so large that it visibly moves the person's clothes, deficient zong qi is indicated. As mentioned, it is likely that the zong qi is related to the chong mai.

From the *Lei Jing* passage previously quoted we can determine that the chong mai ascending the right side of the abdomen and the big luo of the stomach ascending the left side of the abdomen below the breast may be the complementary opposites of the same yin—yang phenomena.

We can think of this idea as reflecting the major energetic connections of the chong mai to the yin and yang organs and the twelve meridians. As the "ocean" of these, the chong mai is their source of nourishment. The zong qi originates from the water and grain qi in the stomach. Perhaps the qi rises from the stomach to the chest to mix with the qi from breathing, becoming zong qi. It then passes downward to the chong mai, from which it is distributed to all the organs and meridians. This possibility is reflected in the comment, "The stomach is the ocean of the five yin and six yang organs."[35] Whether the path of the chong mai is unilateral or bilateral, there is further disagreement about the actual pathway. The *Su Wen* tells us that the chong mai rises up either side of the umbilicus on, or just lateral to, the kidney meridian. The *Nan Jing* posits that it rises parallel to the stomach meridian and surrounds the umbilicus. The *Lei Jing* author describes it as following the kidney meridians from KI-11 to KI-21. According to Li Shi Zhen it ascends between the stomach and kidney meridians.[36] The *Zhen Jiu Ju Ying* seems to settle for the middle ground:

> *The chong mai, du mai and ren mai begin at huiyin {CV-1}. The chong mai stays in the abdomen, passes to henggu {KI-11} and rises up to youmen {KI-21}. All these points are "branching stems" of the kidney meridian. The chong mai runs parallel to the kidney meridian.*[37]

Again, as with qijie and ST-30, we are perhaps safest to consider that the chong mai may be reflected by any of the acupoints from KI-11 to KI-21 and on the area lateral to these points and medial to the stomach meridians.

There is one final, major question regarding the chong mai, concerning the internal branch that the *Ling Shu* describes as ascending in front of the spine.[38] To this, the *Zhen Jiu Jia Yi Jing* author disagrees,[39] feeling that somehow this branch of the chong mai rises up the back. However, no clear statement of what this might involve is given. This idea may be related to the idea from the *Ling Shu* that

BL-11 is the "upper transportation" point of the chong mai.[40] The *Lei Jing* author does agree with the *Ling Shu* statement that this branch ascends deep in the abdomen in front of, and parallel to, the spine.[41] Based on anatomical structures, reason would persuade us to suggest that this branch relates to the aorta or the vena cava. The *Ling Shu* statement that the chong mai ". . . passes blood to the five yin and six yang organs,"[42] and the idea from the *Ling Shu, Tai Su* and Li Shi Zhen that the chong mai is the "blood ocean," support this suggestion.[43] The aorta and vena cava are the two largest blood vessels in the body and might be considered the "blood ocean." This idea may be substantiated and understood in greater depth by examining other early texts.

From studying the internal trajectories of the twelve meridians we know that the heart meridian does not permeate or "belong to" the heart.[44] It permeates the "supporter of the heart," which is probably the aorta or the vena cava and other major blood vessels. The aorta curves down becoming the abdominal aorta that is felt with deeper palpation on the midline of the abdomen. It is also related to the moving qi between the kidneys, and is spoken of in the *Tai Su*, relative to the "blood ocean" and the chong mai. From the following quotation we can begin to understand the major energetic connections of the eight extraordinary vessels, the twelve meridians and the five yin and six yang organs through the source, the root qi of the moving qi between the kidneys:

> *Below the umbilicus is the moving qi between the kidneys, the living energy of the person. This is the root of the twelve meridians. This "blood ocean" {is the} chong mai. This is the ocean of the five yin and six yang organs and the twelve meridians. It nourishes each of the yang and each of the jing; therefore, all the five yin and six yang organs accept it and have it. This moving qi between the kidneys is in the uterus [胞]. The chong mai starts at the inside of the uterus, it is the ocean of the meridians. Now we know that the chong mai causes creation from the moving qi. The lines that go up and down are the chong mai. The line that goes down to the lower parts, the commentary says, "is not the vessel of shao yin."*[45]

The commentary referred to here no longer exists, but must have been in existence before the *Tai Su* was written, circa 610 A.D. From this passage we can understand that the chong mai mediates the actions of the moving qi between the kidneys, the source, in the meridians and organs. It also states the relationship of the moving qi between the kidneys to the "blood ocean": they are one and the same. If, as we have suggested, this is the aorta, these concepts begin to achieve more meaning.

The statement that "it is not the vessel of shao yin" and the *Ling Shu* comment regarding to the "luo vessel of shao yin"[46] may refer to the femoral arteries that branch from the descending aorta, pass through the groin slightly lateral to ST-30 and branch into a number of arteries that travel down to the feet. These pathways are similar to the *Ling Shu* description of the branch of chong mai.

Chong Mai Points

Trajectory	Point	Source
Starts	ST-30	*Su Wen*, Wang Shu He
	CV-1	*Qi Jing Ba Mai Kao* *Zhen Jiu Ju Ying*
Passes	Lateral from KI-11 to KI-21	*Su Wen*, *Nan Jing*, *Qi Jing Ba Mai Kao*
Passes through	KI-11 to KI-21	*Lei Jing* *Zhen Jiu Ju Ying*
Passes to	3 yin foot meridians	*Ling Shu* *Lei Jing*

Chong Mai Trajectory

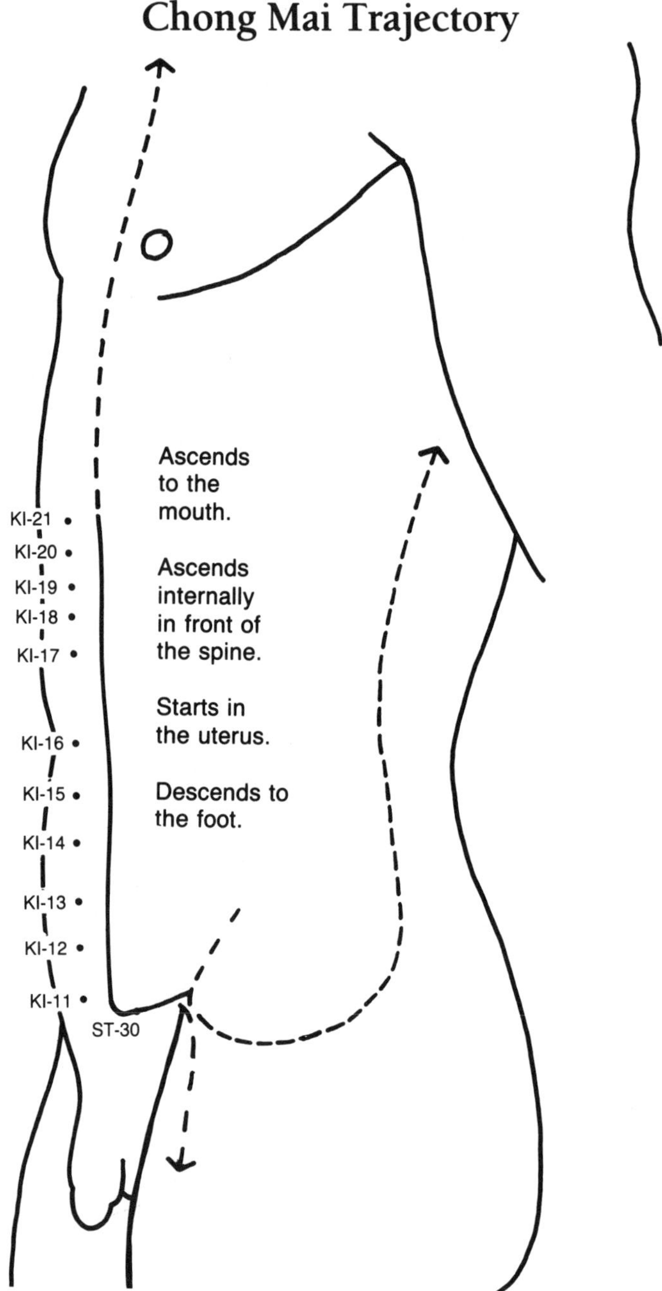

Figure 8

Chong Mai Trajectory

Descending Leg Branch

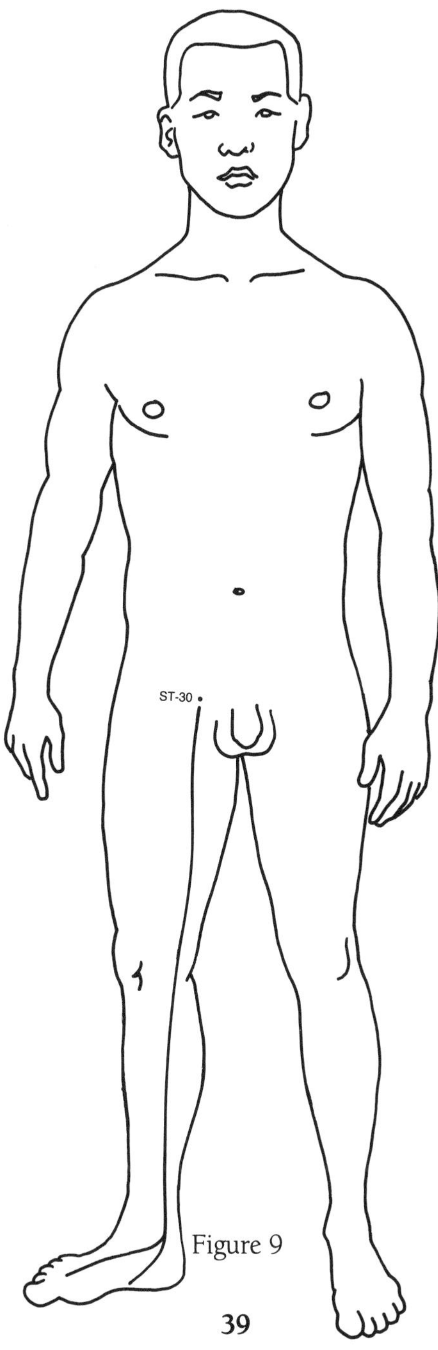

Figure 9

Du Mai

The *Su Wen* says that the du mai or governing vessel:

> *{Starts} in the small abdomen {the kidney reflex area below the umbilicus} and goes down to the center of the pubic bone. In women, it runs down to the hole that is near the urethra {the vagina}.*[47] *The luo [絡] goes around the vagina, passes to the perineum {between the anus and the vagina}, then separates going down to the buttocks, goes down to meet the kidney and bladder meridians inside the upper thighs, rising up the spine and spirally wrapping the kidneys. . .*
>
> *In men, the du mai circulates around the base of the penis and then goes down the center line of the perineum. . .*
>
> *The main vessel starts in the small abdomen, goes up past the umbilicus, up past the heart, enters the throat, comes up to the chin, circulates around the lips and up to the eyes on a line with the pupils.*[48]

The last part of this comment is of particular interest. The "main" vessel rises on the abdomen and not the spine. This trajectory, as we shall see, is often seen as the ren mai. However, this has not attracted much attention from later authors or commentators. In the same chapter, the following comment is made:

> *The du mai and bladder meridian start at jingming {BL-1} and come up over the head. Another branch comes from the lining of the spine, rising up and over the head to the nose.*[49]

The *Ling Shu* comments:

> *The central pulsing {vessel} of the neck is the du mai; it is called fengfu {GV-16}.*[50] *The dividing branch of the du mai is changqiang {GV-1}; it comes up the sides of the spine to the neck and disperses into the head. . . From these ascending lines, a branch is sent out to the scapula bones. Another major branch goes to the bladder meridian and then enters at the side of the spine.*[51]

The *Nan Jing's* description is somewhat clearer:

> *The du mai starts at a point that is below the pole. It comes to the lining of the spine and up to fengfu {GV-16}, entering the brain.*[52]

Wang Shu He comments on this:

> *Below the pole is changqiang {GV-1}. The du mai can control all vessels and becomes like the capital city {central ruler} of the yang vessels.*[53]

The *Nan Jing* itself defines "below the pole" [下極] as the po men [魄門], the anus.[54]

The du mai can be seen to have many trajectories, the main being up the spine. The variations start with the beginning. Ma Shi says, "Changqiang is the luo point of the du mai."[55] However, GV-1 is not always seen as the first point of the du mai. Li Shi Zhen says:

> *Du mai starts at huiyin {CV-1}, going around to the back of the body. It is the ocean of the yang meridians, because it is the controller {of them}.*[56]

Probably, as with the chong mai, it actually starts inside the body, in the abdomen, surfacing at either CV-1 or GV-1, to follow the various trajectories. Wang Bing, who is famous for his eighth century compilations and commentaries on the *Su Wen,* states:

> *Another {branch} starts in the small abdomen, comes up the abdomen, to the center of the eyes, following the path of the ren mai. This is why we can say that the du mai, ren mai and chong mai have different names, but are all the same.*[57]

This is similar to Wang Shu He's idea that each of the vessels has the same source, the same area or point, qijie, ST-30.[58]

The *Ling Shu* says that a branch is "sent out to the scapula bones" from the du mai pathway up the spine.[59] There have been several interpretations of this comment. One commentary says that the du mai "rises up {the spine} and goes out to the bladder meridian and back {to the spine}."[60] The authors of the *Shisi Jing Fa Hui* and the *Zhen Jiu Ju Ying* elucidate this somewhat, stating that it branches from GV-12 to BL-12 and then back to GV-13.[61] The following table presents these variances:

Du Mai Points		
Trajectory	**Point**	**Source**
Starts	GV-1	*Nan Jing*, Wang Shu He
	CV-1	*Qi Jing Ba Mai Kao*
	BL-1	*Su Wen*
	ST-30	Wang Shu He
Passes through	GV-1 to GV-28	most authors
Passes to	BL-12	*Shisi Jing Fa Hui* *Zhen Jiu Ju Ying*
Luo point	GV-1	Ma Shi

Du Mai Trajectory

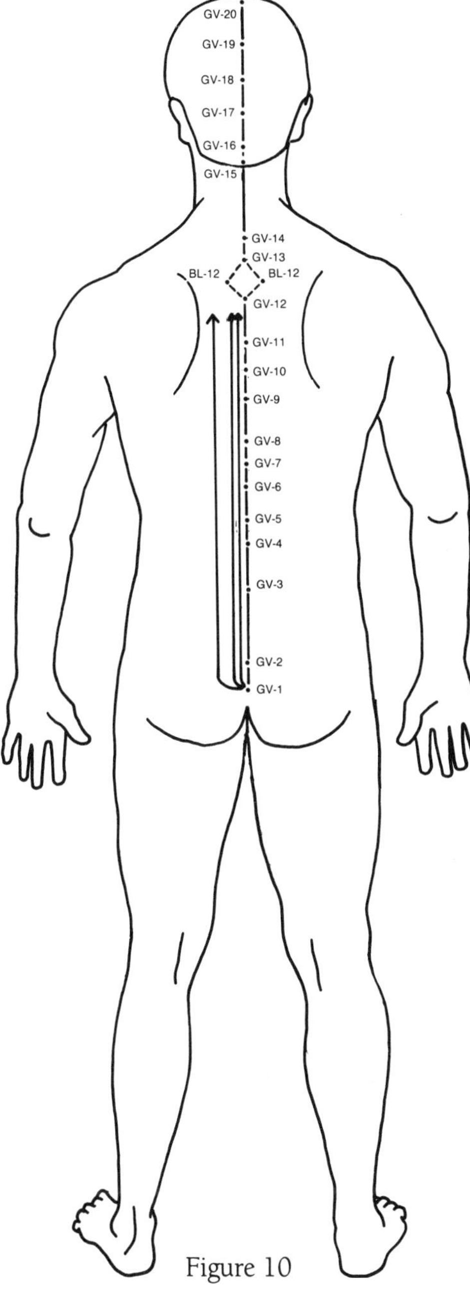

Figure 10

The luo vessels ascend the back from GV-1 in parallel lines

Starts in the uterus, passes to CV-1, GV-1.

The anterior branch follows the ren mai and passes to the genital organs.

The branches ascend either side of the spine.

Du Mai Trajectory

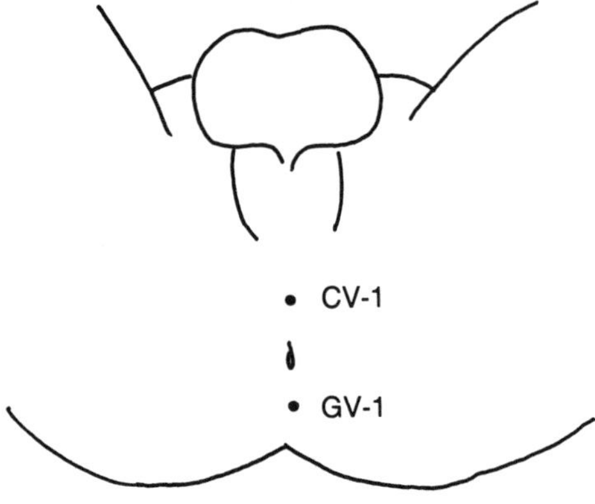

CV-1, GV-1 Location

Figure 11

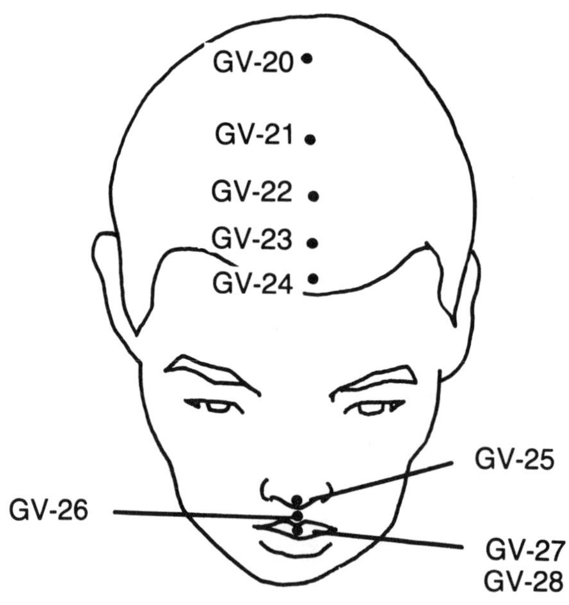

Front of Head Trajectory

Figure 12

Dai Mai

The dai mai has a simple trajectory; most authors agree on the areas through which it passes. The *Su Wen* gives us a theoretical understanding of the dai mai:

> *The Yellow Emperor asked, "Why, when there is weakness of the legs, do we always treat the stomach meridian?"*
>
> *Qi Bo answered, "The chong mai is the ocean of the meridians, the chong mai moistens the valleys. The vessel meets with yang ming {stomach} at the zong muscle. Yin and yang meet at the point qichong {ST-30} which is connected to the zong muscle. The yang ming meridian can control the chong mai and the zong muscle. All these belong to the dai mai. The dai mai goes horizontally around the du mai, so when yang ming is empty, the zong muscle becomes weak; the dai mai cannot pull, and thus the legs become weak. We have to treat the stomach meridian."*[62]

The zong muscle, the "respectable or ancestral muscle," usually refers to the penis in men, and the clitoris in women. It may also refer to the muscles of the abdomen, more particularly the rectus abdominis muscles. We feel that in this discussion Qi Bo is referring to the rectus abdominis rather than the penis. The fundiform ligament, which is continuous with the fascial sheath of the rectus abdominis muscles and the base of the penis, may also be related to the zong muscle.

Mr. Yang explains that the dai character, [帶], means "A belt that when tight commands all the other meridians, controlling by loosening or tightening."[63] The *Ling Shu* tells us more about its trajectory and its relationship to the kidney meridian:

> *The kidney meridian goes behind the knee; it divides, goes to and meets with the bladder meridian. It then rises up and goes to the kidneys and exits belonging to the dai mai.*[64]

The similarity of this trajectory to the internal trajectory of the kidney meridian that passes from KI-16, around the lining of the abdomen to the kidneys, is remarkable, and would confirm the involvement of the dai mai in this trajectory.

The *Nan Jing* offers the following explanation of this trajectory: "The dai mai starts at the rib cage circling the body horizontally."[65] Wang Shu He explains that "at the rib cage" means LV-13.[66] Li Shi Zhen adopts Wang Shu He's comment and explains the trajectory in slightly greater detail:

> *The dai mai starts at the edge of the ribs, which is zhangmen {LV-13}, passing to and circling around daimai {GB-26}, then passing to wushu {GB-27} and weidao {GB-28}.*[67]

The *Zhen Jiu Ju Ying* agrees with this:

> *The dai mai starts 1.8 divisions below the rib cage at daimai, then passes to weidao.*[68]

Dai Mai Points		
Trajectory	**Point**	**Source**
Starts	Rib cage	*Nan Jing*
	LV-13	Wang Shu He, *Qi Jing Ba Mai Kao*
Passes to	GB-26	*Qi Jing Ba Mai Kao, Zhen Jiu Ju Ying*
	GB-27	*Qi Jing Ba Mai Kao*
	GB-28	*Qi Jing Ba Mai Kao, Zhen Jiu Ju Ying*

Dai Mai Trajectory

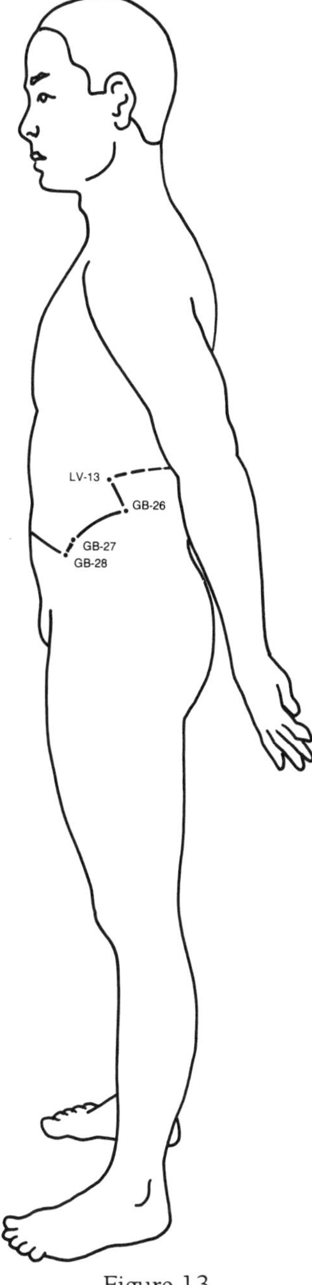

Figure 13

Yin and Yang Qiao Mai

The earliest descriptions of these vessels come from the *Ling Shu*.

> *The qiao vessel divides from the kidney meridian, starts behind the navicular bone and rises to above the internal malleolus. The main vessel of the qiao rises to the inside of the inguinal crease and enters the yin {sexual organs}. Then it rises to the lining of the chest, up to quepen {ST-12}, coming to a point in front of renying {ST-9}, entering the cheek bone and passing up to jingming {BL-1}, meeting the bladder meridian.*[69]
>
> *The yang qiao vessel comes up, the qi of both {the yin and yang qiao} come around {the eyes}, moistening the eyes. If the qi does not nourish them, the eyes will be unable to close.*[69]

The *Ling Shu* tells us more about these relationships:

> *The bladder meridian comes up past the back of the neck and enters the brain, and belongs to the base of the eyes. It is called the "supporter of the eyes." If the head and eyes suffer from problems, treat points on the back of the head between the two muscles {possibly BL-9}. In the brain it divides into two vessels that become the yin qiao and the yang qiao. The yin qiao and yang qiao cross over each other, the yang enters the yin and the yin comes out to the yang and crosses at the sharp edge of the eye. If the qi of the yin qiao mai is excess, the eyes close and cannot open. If the qi of the yang qiao mai is excess, the eyes open and cannot close.*[70]

Ma Shi and the author of the *Lei Jing* both see "the sharp edge of the eye" as the internal canthus.[71] Ma Shi's explanation, that the "yang enters the yin, and the yin comes out to the yang," we may interpret as the yang qiao mai entering the yin, and the yin qiao mai coming out to the yang:

> *The yang qiao mai enters the yin side of the body, the yin qiao mai comes out the yang part of the body and crosses at jingming {BL-1}.*[72]

The idea of the yin coming out to the yang can be understood as the *Ling Shu* idea of the yin qiao mai passing through ST-12, which is a special meeting point of the yang meridians. It is also interesting to note that nerve tracts from one side of the body enter the opposite side of the brain. The nerves cross over in the brain. While this is an interesting parallel, we do not wish to draw any conclusions.

The *Nan Jing* tells us about the qiao mai trajectories:

> *The yang qiao mai begins inside the heel bone, then goes around the external malleolus and rises up to enter feng-chi {GB-20}. . .*
>
> *The yin qiao mai begins inside the heel bone, goes around the internal malleolus and rises to the throat past the chong mai.*[73]

The *Shisi Jing Fa Hui* saw the yin qiao mai as passing from KI-8, to ST-12, to ST-9, to BL-1.[74] The *Zhen Jiu Ju Ying* understood that the pathway only involved KI-6 and KI-8. This text presents the yang qiao mai trajectory in much same way as Li Shi Zhen, except that the pathway includes GB-29.[75] Li Shi Zhen is more detailed in his descriptions of the pathways:

> *The yang qiao mai starts at shenmai {BL-62}, goes to pushen {BL-61}, fuyang {BL-59}, naoshu {SI-10}, jugu {LI-16}, jianyu {LI-15}, renying {ST-9}, dicang {ST-4}, juliao {ST-3}, chengqi {ST-1}, jingming {BL-1}, to end at fengchi {GB-20}. . .*
>
> *The yin qiao mai starts at rangu {KI-2}, goes to zhaohai {KI-6}, jiaoxin {KI-8}, the accumulation point of the yin qiao, to an area in front of renying {ST-9} and above quepen {ST-12}, to jingming {BL-1}.*[76]

Yin Qiao Mai Points		
Trajectory	**Point**	**Source**
Passes through	KI-2	*Qi Jing Ba Mai Kao*
	KI-6	*Zhen Jiu Ju Ying* *Qi Jing Ba Mai Kao*
	KI-8	*Shisi Jing Fa Hui* *Zhen Jiu Ju Ying* *Qi Jing Ba Mai Kao*
	front of ST-9, above ST-12	*Ling Shu* *Qi Jing Ba Mai Kao*
	ST-9	*Shisi Jing Fa Hui*
	ST-12	*Ling Shu, Shisi Jing Fa Hui* *Qi Jing Ba Mai Kao*
	BL-1	*Ling Shu, Shisi Jing Fa Hui* *Qi Jing Ba Mai Kao,* Ma Shi
Accumulation	KI-8	*Qi Jing Ba Mai Kao*

Yang Qiao Mai Points		
Trajectory	**Point**	**Source**
Passes through	BL-1	Ma Shi *Qi Jing Ba Mai Kao* *Zhen Jiu Ju Ying*
	GB-20	*Nan Jing* *Qi Jing Ba Mai Kao*
	BL-62	*Qi Jing Ba Mai Kao* *Zhen Jiu Ju Ying*
	BL-61	*Qi Jing Ba Mai Kao* *Zhen Jiu Ju Ying*
	BL-59	*Qi Jing Ba Mai Kao* *Zhen Jiu Ju Ying*
	SI-10	*Qi Jing Ba Mai Kao* *Zhen Jiu Ju Ying*
	LI-16	*Qi Jing Ba Mai Kao* *Zhen Jiu Ju Ying*
	LI-15	*Qi Jing Ba Mai Kao* *Zhen Jiu Ju Ying*
	ST-9	*Qi Jing Ba Mai Kao* *Zhen Jiu Ju Ying*
	ST-4	*Qi Jing Ba Mai Kao* *Zhen Jiu Ju Ying*
	ST-3	*Qi Jing Ba Mai Kao* *Zhen Jiu Ju Ying*
	ST-1	*Qi Jing Ba Mai Kao* *Zhen Jiu Ju Ying*
	GB-29	*Zhen Jiu Ju Ying*

Yin Qiao Mai Trajectory

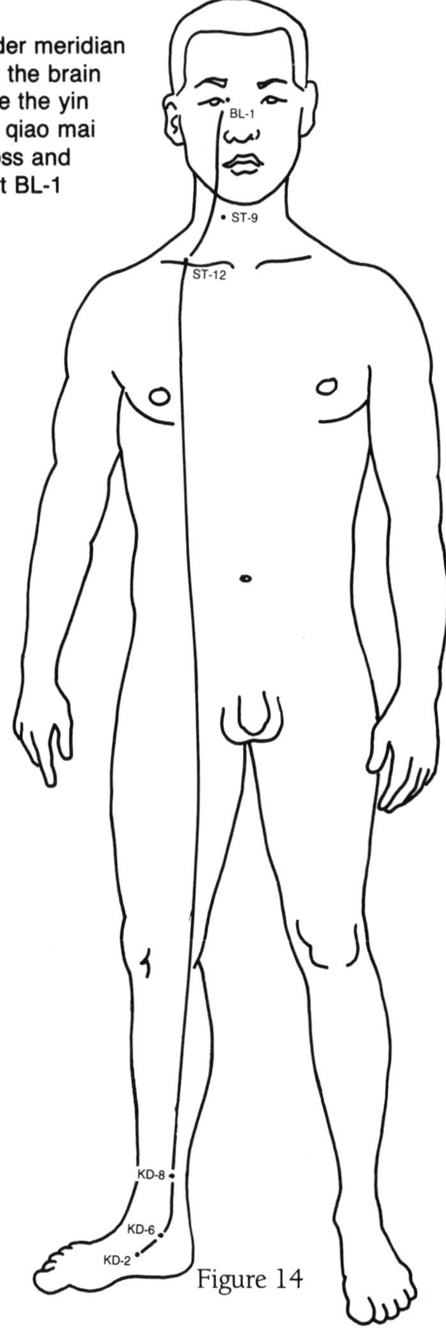
The bladder meridian
divides in the brain
to become the yin
and yang qiao mai
which cross and
emerge at BL-1
BL-1
ST-9
ST-12
KD-8
KD-6
KD-2

Figure 14

Yang Qiao Mai Trajectory

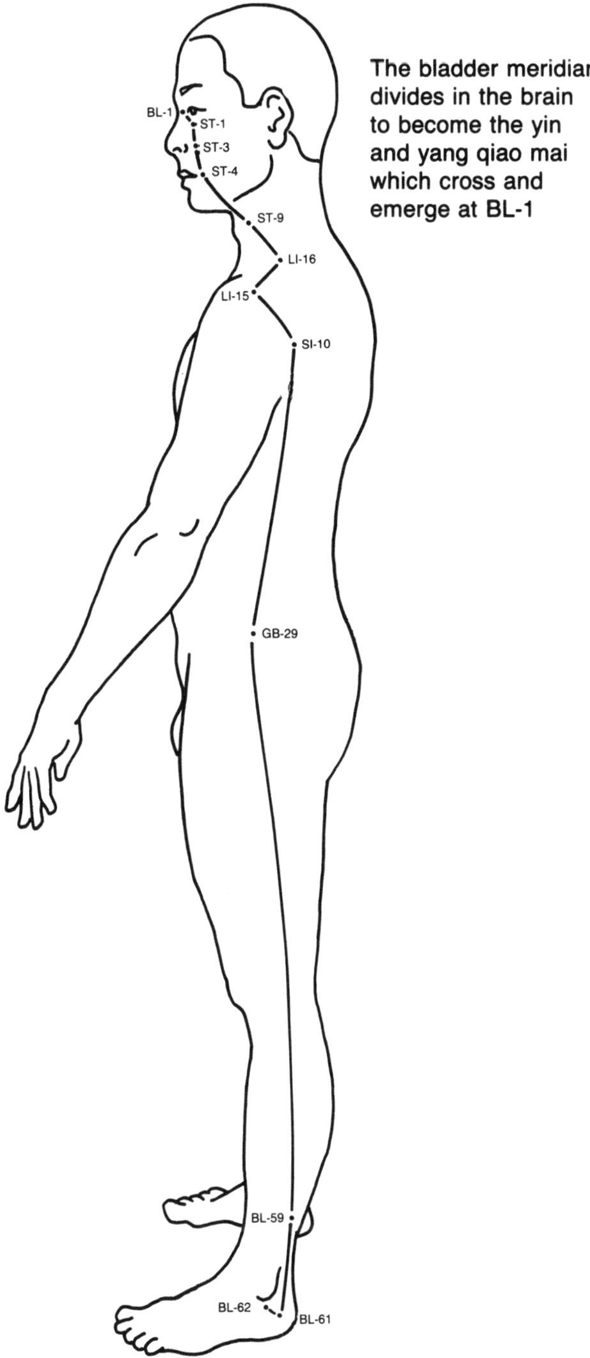

Figure 15

Yin and Yang Wei Mai

The *Su Wen* discusses the yang wei mai in a chapter on lumbar pain:

> *For symptoms of swelling and pain on the lumbar area, or irritability and a swollen spot on the painful area, insert the needle into the vessel of the yang wei. The place {to treat} is on the external aspect of the leg, ten divisions above the bottom of the heel, where it meets the tai yang.*[77]

The *Tai Su* states that this point may be GB-35, since the name is yangjiao, "yang crossing."[78] The same chapter of the *Su Wen* describes lumbar pain and treatment of the yin wei mai:

> *Lumbar pain caused by the fei yang {flying yang} vessel has swelling on the painful spot or irritability with pain. If it gets worse, people become afraid and sad. For lumbar pain of this nature, insert a needle five divisions above the internal malleolus. This is the point of fei yang, in front of the kidney meridian, at the meeting place of the yin wei mai.*[79]

Some of the writing at this time, 100-300 B.C., was strangely worded making comprehension difficult. Feiyang, flying yang [飛陽] is the point BL-58, the luo point of the bladder meridian. Quite possibly, the flying yang vessel is the luo vessel of the bladder meridian. Etymologically, the character fei [飛] is derived from the image of a bird flapping its wings. It connotes the dividing of left and right.[80] Although it is the name of the point BL-58, the term fei yang could refer to the dividing of left and right parts of the yang. This function of dividing the left and right parts of the body is part of the general function of the yin and yang wei mai. According to the *Zhen Jiu Jia Yi Jing*, the acupoint five divisions above the internal malleolus in front of the kidney meridian, which meets the yin wei mai, is KI-9.[81]

Regarding the trajectories of the wei mai the *Nan Jing* posits:

> *The yang wei starts at the meeting of the yang meridians. The yin wei starts at the yin crossing.*[82]

Li Shi Zhen says that this "yin crossing" is zhubin (KI-9),[83] and quotes from Wang Qi Xuan that the yang wei starts at chengshan {BL-57}.[84] Li Shi Zhen himself proposes a complex trajectory for the yin and yang wei mai:

> *The yin wei mai starts at the crossing of the yin at zhubin {KI-9}, the accumulation point of the yin wei, five divisions above the internal malleolus. It rises to the center of the muscle {of the thigh?}, enters the small abdomen, meets the spleen, liver, kidney and stomach meridians at fushe {SP-13}, meets the spleen meridian at daheng {SP-15} and fuai {SP-16}, goes to the side to meet the liver meridian at qimen {LV-14}, goes past the diaphragm, up the chest, up the sides of the throat, meeting the ren mai at tiantu {CV-22} and lianquan {CV-23}, rising to finish on the forehead.*[85]
>
> *The yang wei mai starts at the meeting of each yang, the point is jinmen {BL-63}. It comes to yangjiao {GB-35}, the yang crossing point and accumulation point of the yang wei mai, rises up the sides of the small abdomen, goes to juliao {GB-29}, up the sides of the ribcage to the shoulder where it meets the large intestine, bladder and small intestine at binao {LI-14}, then ascends the front of the shoulder to naohui {TW-13} and tianliao {TW-15}. Then it meets the gallbladder, triple warmer and stomach at jianjing {GB-21}, goes to the back of the shoulder, meets the yang qiao mai and large intestine at naoshu {SI-10}, goes behind the ears to meet the triple warmer and gallbladder at fengchi {GB-20}. Then it goes to naokong {GB-19}, chengling {GB-18}, zhengying {GB-17}, muchuang {GB-16}, linqi {GB-15} and to the forehead where it meets the five vessels of the gallbladder, triple warmer, large intestine, stomach and yang wei at yangbai {GB-14}. Then it goes to the ear to benshen {GB-13}.*[86]

The location of LV-14 used by Li Shi Zhen is two ribs below the nipples, between the ribs.

Much of this description is probably derived from earlier sources. The *Shisi Jing Fa Hui* presents the yang wei trajectory thus:

> *BL-63, GB-35, GB-29, LI-14, SI-10, TW-15, GB-21 GV-15, GV-16, GB-20, GB-19, GB-18, GB-17, GB-16, GB-15, GB-14, GB-13.*[87]

The trajectory of the yin wei mai is identical to Li Shi Zhen's description. The *Zhen Jiu Ju Ying* offers the following for the wei mai trajectories:

> *Yang wei mai: BL-63, GB-35, SI-10, TW-15, GB-21, GB-14 to GB-13, GB-15, GB-17, GB-19, GB-20, GV-16, GV-15.*
>
> *Yin wei mai: KI-9, SP-16, SP-15, SP-13, LV-14, CV-22, CV-23.*[88]

These trajectories are all sufficiently similar to justify area and point correspondences.

Yin Wei Points		
Trajectory	**Point**	**Source**
Passes through	KI-9	*Qi Jing Ba Mai Kao* *Shisi Jing Fa Hui* *Zhen Jiu Ju Ying*
	SP-13	*Qi Jing Ba Mai Kao* *Shisi Jing Fa Hui* *Zhen Jiu Ju Ying*
	SP-15	*Qi Jing Ba Mai Kao* *Shisi Jing Fa Hui* *Zhen Jiu Ju Ying*
	SP-16	*Qi Jing Ba Mai Kao* *Shisi Jing Fa Hui* *Zhen Jiu Ju Ying*
	LV-14	*Qi Jing Ba Mai Kao* *Shisi Jing Fa Hui* *Zhen Jiu Ju Ying*
	CV-22	*Qi Jing Ba Mai Kao* *Shisi Jing Fa Hui* *Zhen Jiu Ju Ying*
	CV-23	*Qi Jing Ba Mai Kao* *Shisi Jing Fa Hui* *Zhen Jiu Ju Ying*

Yang Wei Mai Points		
Trajectory	**Point**	**Source**
Passes through	BL-57	*Qi Jing Ba Mai Kao*
	BL-63	*Qi Jing Ba Mai Kao, Shisi Jing Fa Hui Zhen Jiu Ju Ying*
	GB-35	*Qi Jing Ba Mai Kao, Shisi Jing Fa Hui Zhen Jiu Ju Ying*
	GB-29	*Qi Jing Ba Mai Kao*
	LI-14	*Qi Jing Ba Mai Kao, Shisi Jing Fa Hui*
	TW-13	*Qi Jing Ba Mai Kao*
	TW-15	*Qi Jing Ba Mai Kao, Shisi Jing Fa Hui Zhen Jiu Ju Ying*
	GB-21	*Qi Jing Ba Mai Kao, Shisi Jing Fa Hui Zhen Jiu Ju Ying*
	SI-10	*Qi Jing Ba Mai Kao, Shisi Jing Fa Hui Zhen Jiu Ju Ying*
	GB-20	*Qi Jing Ba Mai Kao, Shisi Jing Fa Hui Zhen Jiu Ju Ying*
	GB-19	*Qi Jing Ba Mai Kao, Shisi Jing Fa Hui Zhen Jiu Ju Ying*
	GB-18	*Qi Jing Ba Mai Kao Shisi Jing Fa Hui*
	GB-17	*Qi Jing Ba Mai Kao, Shisi Jing Fa Hui Zhen Jiu Ju Ying*
	GB-16	*Qi Jing Ba Mai Kao, Shisi Jing Fa Hui Zhen Jiu Ju Ying*
	GB-15	*Qi Jing Ba Mai Kao, Shisi Jing Fa Hui Zhen Jiu Ju Ying*
	GB-14	*Qi Jing Ba Mai Kao, Shisi Jing Fa Hui Zhen Jiu Ju Ying*
	GB-13	*Qi Jing Ba Mai Kao, Shisi Jing Fa Hui Zhen Jiu Ju Ying*
	GV-15	*Shisi Jing Fa Hui Zhen Jiu Ju Ying*
	GV-16	*Shisi Jing Fa Hui Zhen Jiu Ju Ying*

Yin Wei Mai Trajectory

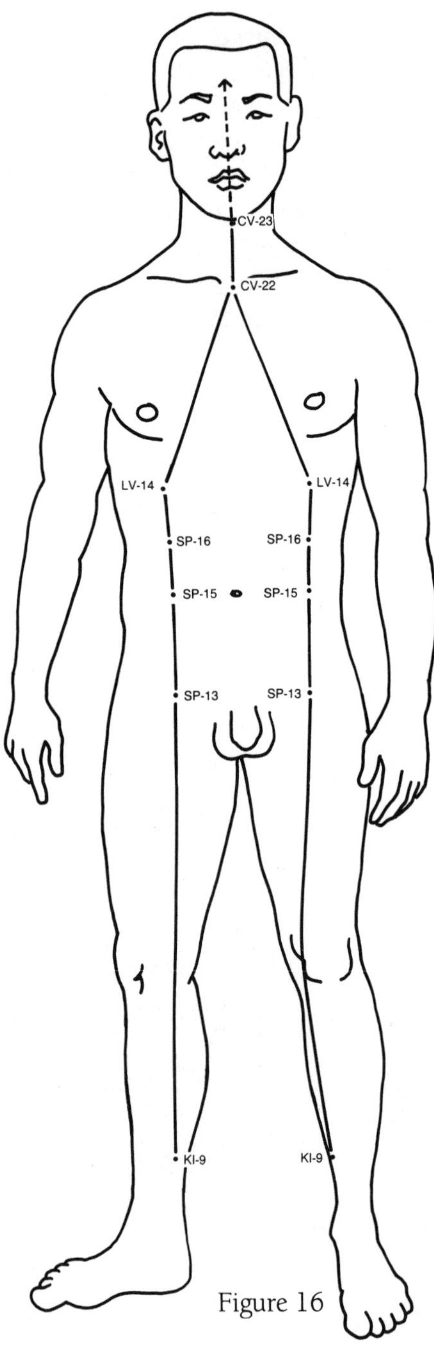

Figure 16

Yang Wei Mai Trajectory

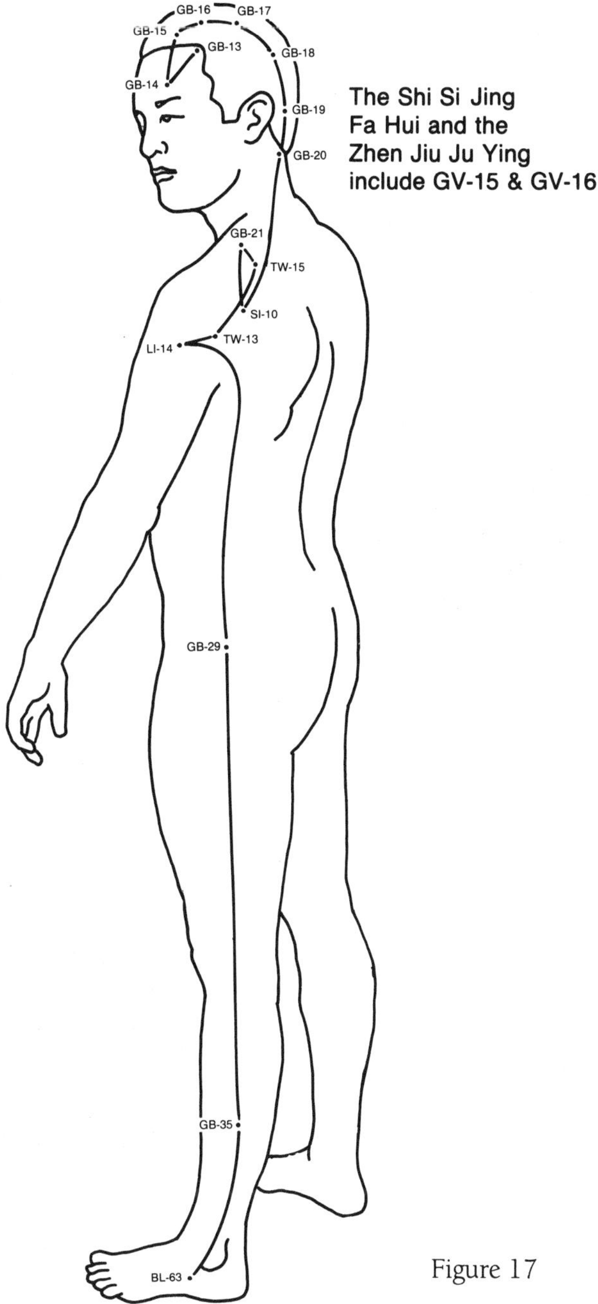

The Shi Si Jing Fa Hui and the Zhen Jiu Ju Ying include GV-15 & GV-16.

Figure 17

Applications of Extraordinary Vessel Theory

This present study of the eight extraordinary vessels is by no means exhaustive. There are undoubtedly variations and descriptions that we have not recorded. However, those presented do include sufficient information for practical application. As students of Oriental medicine we cannot simply accept one theory and forget the rest. Understanding the generality of the descriptions, particularly the "standard" descriptions that we create as organizational aids, we should be aware of many of these possible pathways. When we palpate a point and find reactiveness, or observe signs and symptoms in an area, it may be a non-standard idea or variant trajectory that provides the clue with which we are able to solve the problem. If we know only one possibility, we diminish our chances of making a complete differential diagnosis. It is always useful (unhappily or interestingly so, depending on one's perspective), to remember that each of these trajectories are just theories. It is inevitable that events in a living human will confound theory. As a working whole, the body is greater than the sum of the theories used to describe the various parts. The greater our background knowledge, the greater our chances of helping any patient.

It is in treatment that a broad knowledge of theory and diagnosis is particularly useful. Information regarding the eight extraordinary vessels provides us with a wide range of point correspondences and potential energetic results. Certainly, the trajectories of the vessels demonstrate that considerable energetic exchange and transformation occurs in the abdomen, at the energetic center that we described. Four of the extraordinary vessels have their origins on, or in, the abdomen. The other four pass over or around the edges. These paths represent the simplest and most obvious level of energetics involved. There are other deeper energetic functions.

The following tables summarize the pathway discussions. As well as broadening our diagnostic repertoire, they further serve as potential treatment points, following the *Zhen Jiu Da Cheng's* principle:

> *One has to examine the right and left, upper and lower {parts of the body}. . . feel and palpate the body to find something with your hands, then do some exercises and*

> *take the disease away with the {eight} points. This is the rule, according to the rule, one can remove diseases. If the diseases don't pass, one has to ask {palpate} the meeting points {and treat them}.*[89]

If the regular treatment doesn't work, treat the meeting points on the pathways of the vessels. As we will see in the next chapter, the meeting points are probably the "he" points located around the elbows and knees. The *Zhen Jiu Ju Ying* seems clearly to refer to the he points, but in the *Zhen Jiu Da Cheng,* the reference is not so clear, the "meeting" points are just as likely intended.

Extraordinary Vessel Meeting or Correspondence Points

The following tables summarize the points that are associated with the eight extraordinary vessels. Palpation and observation of these points is a significant key to the successful use of the extraordinary vessels. Some of the points listed are associated with the twelve meridians or other energetic entities. We have included these as they may be useful. However, correspondence points of the main trajectories are likely more useful.

Palpation is best done using the pads of the thumbs. First apply gentle pressure, then firmer pressure, to confirm the absence or presence of reactions such as pressure pain, tightness, tension, swelling, looseness, puffiness. Palpation along the length of the ren mai can reflect the condition of the ren mai. The abdominal and chest trajectories of the ren mai may possibly, but not certainly, reflect the du mai as well.

Abdominal Points	
Point	**Indication**
CV-1	chong mai, du mai
CV-5	ming men, triple warmer
CV-7	triple warmer, bladder, gallbladder, chong mai, du mai.
CV-10	spleen
CV-12	lung, triple warmer, stomach
CV-22	yin wei mai
CV-23	yin wei mai.
ST-30	du mai, ren mai, chong mai and possibly the zong qi
ST-12	yin qiao mai
KI-11 to KI-21	chong mai
LV-13	dai mai.
LV-14	yin wei mai.
SP-13	spleen, liver, kidney, stomach, yin wei mai.
SP-15	yin wei mai
SP-16	yin wei mai

Note that the area between the kidney and stomach meridians from KI-11 to KI-21 also reflects the chong mai.

Leg Points	
Point	**Indication**
KI-2	yin qiao mai
KI-6	yin qiao mai
KI-8	yin qiao mai
KI-9	yin wei mai
BL-57	yang wei mai
BL-58	possibly yin wei mai
BL-59	yang qiao mai
BL-61	yang qiao mai
BL-62	yang qiao mai
BL-63	yang wei mai.
GB-29	yang wei mai, yang qiao mai.
GB-35	yang wei mai

Arm and Shoulder Points	
Point	**Indication**
LI-14	large intestine, bladder, stomach, yang wei mai
LI-15	yang qiao mai
LI-16	yang qiao mai
TW-13	yang wei mai
TW-15	yang wei mai
GB-21	gallbladder, triple warmer, stomach, yang wei mai
SI-10	yang wei & yang qiao mai (large intestine).

All points on the du mai will reflect the condition of the du mai, especially GV-12, GV-13 and GV-14.

Points on the Head, Neck, Back, Side	
Point	**Indication**
GV-1	ren mai
GV-15	yang wei mai
GV-16	yang wei mai
CV-24	large intestine, stomach, du mai
BL-1	du mai, yin qiao mai, yang qiao mai
BL-12	du mai
GB-13	yang wei mai
GB-14	yang wei mai, gallbladder, triple warmer, large intestine & stomach
GB-15	yang wei mai
GB-16	yang wei mai
GB-17	yang wei mai
GB-18	yang wei mai
GB-19	yang wei mai
GB-20	yang wei & yang qiao mai, triple warmer, gallbladder
GB-26	dai mai
GB-27	dai mai
GB-28	dai mai
ST-1	yang qiao mai, ren mai
ST-3	yang qiao mai
ST-4	yang qiao mai
ST-9	yang qiao mai, yin qiao mai

Notes

[1] Modern Chinese research regarding the meridian concept is just beginning to appear in English. The *Jingluo Phenomena*, Volume One, demonstrates the pathways through dermatologic illnesses. The second volume in that series describes meridian traces through stimulus and other means. English editions of this material are in the process of translation at this time.

[2] *Su Wen*, Chapter 60, p. 319.

[3] *Ling Shu*, Chapter 65, p. 463.

[4] *Lei Jing*, p. 280.

[5] *Nei Jing Jie Po Sheng Li Xue*, pp. 110-111 *passim*.

[6] *Huang Di Nei Jing Tai Su*, p. 145.

[7] Li Shi Zhen, *Qi Jing Ba Mai Kao*, vol. 1, pp. 18-19.

[8] *Ibid.*

[9] *Ibid.*

[10] *Nan Jing*, Chapter 28, vol. 2, p. 14, *passim*.

[11] *Ling Shu*, Chapter 10, p. 145.

[12] *Su Wen*, Chapter 60, p. 319.

[13] *Ling Shu*, Chapter 38, pp. 308-9

[14] *Lei Jing*, from the *Nei Jing Jie Po Sheng Li Xue*, *passim*.

[15] *Ling Shu*, Chapter 62, p. 434.

[16] *Ibid.*, Chapter 65, p. 463.

[17] *Ibid.*, Chapter 33, pp. 281-282.

[18] *Nan Jing*, Chapter 28, vol. 2, p. 14.

[19] Wang Shu He, *Commentary on the Nan Jing*, Chapter 28, vol. 2, pp. 14-15.

[20] *Ibid.*

[21] Wang Shu He, *Mai Jing*, vol. 2, p. 16.

[22] *Morohashi Encyclopedic Dictionary*.

[23] *Fujido's Etymological Dictionary*.

[24] *Ling Shu*, Chapter 52, p. 390.

[25] *Ibid., passim.*

[26] Li Shi Zhen, *Qi Jing Ba Mai Kao* quoted from *Nei Jing Jie Po Sheng Li Xue*, p. 115, and the *Zhen Jiu Ju Ying*, pp. 133-4 *passim.*

[27] *Ling Shu*, Chapter 62.

[28] *Ibid.*, Chapter 65.

[29] *Huang Di Nei Jing Tai Su*, vol. 10, p. 153, *passim.*

[30] *Ling Shu*, Chapter 75, p. 543.

[31] *Zhen Jiu Jia Yi Jing*, from the *Nei Jing Jie Po Sheng Li Xue*, p. 117.

[32] Li Shi Zhen, *Qi Jing Ba Mai Kao*, from *Nei Jing Jie Po Sheng Li Xue*, p. 115.

[33] *Lei Jing*, quoted from the *Nei Jing Jie Po Sheng Li Xue*, p. 117.

[34] *Su Wen*, Chapter 18, p. 111.

[35] *Ibid.*, Chapter 29, p. 181 *passim*, and *Ling Shu* Chapter 62, p. 431 *passim.*

[36] *Su Wen*, Chapter 60 p. 319; *Nan Jing*, Chapter 28, vol. 2, p. 14; *Lei Jing*, p. 280; Li Shi Zhen, *Qi Jing Ba Mai Kao*, from *Nei Jing Jie Po Sheng Li Xue*, p. 115.

[37] *Zhen Jiu Ju Ying*, pp. 133-134.

[38] *Ling Shu*, Chapter 65.

[39] *Zhen Jiu Jia Yi Jing*, p. 117 of the *Nei Jing Jie Po Sheng Li Xue*, *passim.*

[40] *Ling Shu*, Chapter 33, p. 281 *passim.*

[41] *Lei Jing*, from p. 115 of the *Nei Jing Jie Po Sheng Li Xue*, *passim.*

[42] *Ling Shu*, Chapter 38, p. 308.

[43] *Ibid.*, Chapter 33, p. 281; *Huang Di Nei Jing Tai Su,* vol. 10, p. 153; and Li Shi Zhen, *Qi Jing Ba Mai Kao,* vol. 1 p. 12.

[44] See the discussion of the internal trajectories of the twelve meridians in *Hara: Reflections on the Sea.*

[45] *Huang Di Nei Jing Tai Su,* vol. 10, p. 153.

[46] *Ling Shu,* Chapter 38.

[47] Zhang Zhi Zong saw this as the vagina. See p. 120 of the *Nei Jing Jie Po Sheng Li Xue.*

[48] *Su Wen,* Chapter 60, p. 320.

[49] *Ibid.*, pp. 320-321.

[50] *Ling Shu* Chapter 2, p. 26,

[51] *Ibid.*, Chapter 10, p. 145.

[52] *Nan Jing,* Chapter 28, vol. 2, p. 14.

[53] Wang Shu He, *Commentary on the Nan Jing,* vol. 2, p. 14.

[54] *Nan Jing,* Chapter 44, vol. 3, p. 10.

[55] Ma Shi, quoted from p. 121 of *Nei Jing Jie Po Sheng Li Xue.*

[56] Li Shi Zhen, *Qi Jing Ba Mai Kao,* quoted from the *Nei Jing Jie Po Sheng Li Xue,* p. 120.

[57] Wang Bing quoted from p. 121 of the *Nei Jing Jie Po Sheng Li Xue.*

[58] Wang Shu He, *Commentary on the Nan Jing,* vol. 2, pp. 14-15, *passim.*

[59] *Ling Shu,* Chapter 10, p. 145.

[60] Ma Shi, quoted from the *Nei Jing Jie Po Sheng Li Xue,* p. 121.

[61] *Shisi Jing Fa Hui,* p. 163 *passim. Zhen Jiu Ju Ying,* p. 117 *passim.*

[62] *Su Wen,* Chapter 44, pp. 248-249.

[63] Mr. Yang, quoted from p. 128 of the *Nei Jing Jie Po Sheng Li Xue.*

[64] *Ling Shu,* Chapter 11, p. 149.

[65] *Nan Jing,* Chapter 28, vol. 2, p. 15.

[66] Wang Shu He, *Commentary on the Nan Jing*, vol. 2, p. 15.

[67] Li Shi Zhen, *Qi Jing Ba Mai Kao*, vol. 1, p. 23 *passim*.

[68] *Zhen Jiu Ju Ying*, p. 135.

[69] *Ling Shu*, Chapter 17, p. 190.

[70] *Ibid.* Chapter 21, p. 215.

[71] *Nei Jing Jie Po Sheng Li Xue*, p. 135.

[72] *Ibid.*

[73] *Nan Jing*, Chapter 28, vol. 2, pp. 15-16.

[74] *Shisi Jing Fa Hui*, p. 183 *passim*.

[75] *Zhen Jiu Ju Ying*, p. 133 *passim*.

[76] Li Shi Zhen, *Qi Jing Ba Mai Kao*, vol. 1, pp. 7-8 *passim*.

[77] *Su Wen*, Chapter 41, p. 230.

[78] *Huang Di Nei Jing Tai Su*, vol. 10, p. 155.

[79] *Su Wen* Chapter 41, p. 230.

[80] *Fujido's Etymological Dictionary*.

[81] *Nei Jing Jie Po Sheng Li Xue*, p. 143.

[82] *Nan Jing*, Chapter 28, vol. 2, p. 16.

[83] Li Shi Zhen, *Qi Jing Ba Mai Kao*, vol. 1, p. 2.

[84] *Ibid*, p. 6.

[85] *Ibid.*, p. 2.

[86] *Ibid.*, p. 3.

[87] *Shisi Jing Fa Hui*, p. 185 *passim*.

[88] *Zhen Jiu Ju Ying*, pp. 134-135, *passim*.

[89] *Zhen Jiu Da Cheng*, p. 191.

Extraordinary Vessels

Classical Symptoms and Treatments of the Extraordinary Vessels

The texts discussing the symptoms that indicate problems treated by the extraordinary vessels are the same texts that developed their theory and pathways: the *Nan Jing*, Wang Shu He's *Commentary on the Nan Jing* and the *Zhen Jing Zhi Nan, Acupuncture South Pointer*. Much of this last book is repeated in the *Zhen Jiu Ju Ying, Gathering of Eminent Acupuncturists* and the *Zhen Jiu Da Cheng, Compendium of Acupuncture and Moxibustion*. There are also basic symptomologies in the *Su Wen* and *Ling Shu*. The symptom descriptions in the *Zhen Jing Zhi Nan*, *Zhen Jiu Ju Ying* and *Zhen Jiu Da Cheng* are listed according to the points used. The *Zhen Jing Zhi Nan* and *Zhen Jiu Ju Ying* list symptoms for each point pair with suggestions·of the twelve meridians usually associated with each symptom, and suggest treating the "he" points of these meridians where appropriate. In the *Zhen Jiu Da Cheng* there are symptom lists for single points and for pairs of points, and lists of diseases and symptom patterns treatable by the eight master points in combination with other points. These point combinations, which address both the root and local levels of the condition, are suitable for specific problems, and expand the clinical use of the extraordinary vessels.

A few of the extraordinary vessel symptoms described by Li Shi Zhen, where he indicated the use of acupuncture, have been included, though his treatment style was predominantly herbal, with some adjunctive acupuncture. While Li Shi Zhen did use some acupuncture to treat the extraordinary vessels, he had a different view than the author of the *Zhen Jiu Da Quan*. He did not, for example, use the eight master points we use today. However, his mastery of extraordinary vessel theory is clear and practical consideration should be given to his treatment ideas.

Diagnostic Methods

Some of the signs listed by the texts are determined or verified by palpation. Most modern practitioners use palpation to find pressure pain, tension, tightness, looseness, swelling, flaccidity, weakness, knots or lack of elasticity. When palpating, it is best to use the fingers to steady the hand and palpate with the thumbs. Always strive to be consistent. Begin with gentle pressure and if no reaction is elicited, employ firmer pressure to confirm that the point is not reactive.[1] In the older texts cryptic suggestions to "investigate the ren mai," or any of the extraordinary vessels, or to "choose a point," become more useful when interpreted as instructions to palpate the meridian pathway.

The lists of symptoms for each of the vessels include indications; from these it is obvious that treating these vessels has a broad effect. Many problems may be treated using the few points described. These lists of indications also demonstrate the physical and structural effects of extraordinary vessel treatments. For example, the du mai treats rigidity of the spine; the dai mai treats an imbalance of one side of the body from the ribs down to the legs; the yin and yang qiao mai treat relative tension and looseness of the medial and lateral aspects of the legs. The yang qiao mai also treats tightness of the lumbar area and back when bending and a feeling of fullness or swelling on one side of the body. The topological nature of the extraordinary vessels has been recognized for a long time.

It is useful to combine the symptomology of the vessels with palpatory diagnosis and topological relationships. Palpation was recommended by the *Zhen Jing Zhi Nan, Zhen Jiu Ju Ying* and *Zhen Jiu Da Cheng,* among other books. These instruct us to examine the upper, lower, left and right parts. However, these books give us no clear or systematic description of the palpatory and topological relationships to use. Modern practitioners such as Dr. Manaka and Mr. Ito do give clear descriptions that help us understand the older books.

Another addition to the diagnostic information of the extraordinary vessels are the "meeting" or "correspondence" points on their pathways. These are the points that describe, as Dr. Manaka says, "the dividing lines of the body," and have great diagnostic and therapeutic usefulness. As the *Zhen Jiu Da Cheng* states:

> *One has to examine the right and left, upper and lower {parts of the body}. . . Feel and palpate the body to find something with your hands, then do some exercises and take the disease away with the {eight} points. This is the rule, according to the rule, one can remove diseases. If the diseases do not pass, one has to ask {palpate} the meeting points {and treat them}. . .*[2]

The meeting points discussed could be interpreted as either the he points, found around the elbows and knees, or the meeting points of the extraordinary vessels. The same character is used in either case. Given the context of this discussion from the *Da Cheng*, it is more likely that this rule refers to the extraordinary vessel meeting points. However, similar discussions in the *Zhen Jing Zhi Nan* and *Zhen Jiu Ju Ying* make more sense when seen as referring to the he points, becoming more obvious in context:

> *Make the upper and lower parts connect, make {the patient} comfortable, taking away the suffering or pain.*[3]

Dr. Manaka's treatment procedures clearly adopt these recommendations. He uses palpatory diagnosis; he also uses therapeutic exercises. He connects the upper and lower parts using the extraordinary vessels and emphasizes the importance of the patient's comfort and relaxation during treatment. The meeting points are a further step in his treatment style that may be used as required. This treatment model is easy to use and has the advantage of approaching the problem from a variety of different directions.

Treatment Techniques

When treatments for the extraordinary vessels were described in the old books, there were, unfortunately, few descriptions of the needle or moxa techniques recommended. In the *Zhen Jiu Da Cheng*, for example, there are descriptions of needle and moxa techniques for tonification and dispersion, but no indication that these techniques are to be applied to the extraordinary vessel points. Since there is no reference to tonifying or dispersing the eight points, knowing exactly what needle technique to use is difficult. Similar difficulties are encountered when examining the polarity of needle application. Most texts refer to inserting the master point first, then the coupled point. However, it is not clear whether this is done bilaterally, contralaterally or ipsilaterally. There are some hints that the needles should be oriented according to the side of the body affected, location of the problem or according to what is found by palpation of the "right, left, upper and lower parts."[4] It seems that both classical and modern practitioners had their own treatment approach to the extraordinary vessels. Most seem to use some idea of polarity or topology, but these were not always clearly defined.

The use of the extraordinary vessel points in combination with other body points also varies according to different authors. The *Zhen Jing Zhi Nan*, which first described the eight points, and the

Zhen Jiu Ju Ying, which reiterated the *Zhi Nan* treatments, both specify treating the master points first followed by the coupled points. Selection of the master point was presumably determined by the examination of symptom complexes and possibly oriented according to the findings of palpation or the location of the problem. Once the points were inserted, both texts specify "Dao Yin," Daoist breathing exercises.[5] Then, if the problem was not cured, the practitioner was advised to select the corresponding he points. When the patient was comfortable and relaxed, the needles were removed.[6] Presumably, the he points were selected from the meridians that corresponded to each symptom. For example, SP-4, which indicates the chong mai, was related to these symptoms:[7]

Symptoms	**Meridians**
nine kinds of heart pain	heart, stomach
diarrhea that won't stop	large intestine, stomach
umbilicus and abdomen swollen and painful	triple warmer, stomach

To clarify these relationships we can conceptualize these correspondences as "sets":

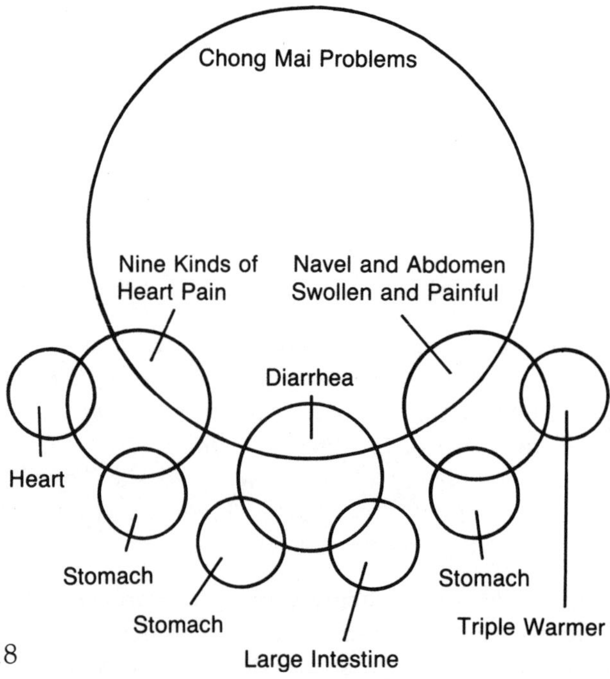

Figure 18

All the symptoms belong to the larger, more general set of conditions that may be treated through the chong mai. Each is also a member of a subset of conditions related to a particular meridian that could be treated through the chong mai, the particular meridian he points or both. Gao Wu, the author of the *Zhen Jiu Ju Ying*, summarizes this idea with a simple analogy:

> *If we think about this treatment style, it is really broad, it's like trying to catch a single rabbit in a field with a massive net.*[8]

The extraordinary vessel is the massive net, the symptom the rabbit. To continue the analogy, we can imagine the associated meridian he point as a hand net. This series of correspondences is historically interesting as these were possibly influential for the later development of differential diagnosis, symptom complexes and point selection.

There are no clear statements of the treatment techniques employed. We can only recommend the insertion of needles to the needle depths generally specified for each acupoint. However, in the *Zhen Jiu Da Cheng*, the approach is different. When treating just the extraordinary vessel points, the *Da Cheng* specifies treating the master point first, then the coupled point. The decisions regarding which point was to be the master point and what would be the polarity of the treatment seems to have been made in a manner similar to that described in the *Zhi Nan* and *Ju Ying*. However, the *Zhen Jiu Da Cheng* describes symptom complexes with specific sets of treatments that combine the extraordinary vessel points with other body points. These combinations always require treatment of the master point followed by the rest of the points in sequence. In other words, it seems to have been the experience of *Da Cheng* author that the master point in combination with the other body points was sufficient, the coupled points were not necessary.

When treating just the extraordinary vessel points, the *Da Cheng* refers to exercises, though not specifically Dao Yin exercise, followed by treatment of the he points. However, we believe this reference to the he points implies the correspondence or meeting points of the eight extraordinary vessels rather than the meridian he points. In short, be aware of the treatment considerations of the source. The style associated with the *Da Cheng* is an essential, if not totally clear, element of the information. Note also that occasionally a point will appear twice in the *Da Cheng* lists of points. This seems to indicate that the points are to be treated in sequence with in-and-out needle techniques and not simultaneously while retaining the needles. Examine the main effects of the points given in the *Da Cheng* descriptions. The four yin points treat mainly organ, deeper, more yin problems. The four yang points treat mainly non-organ, superficial, yang problems.

Regarding needle and moxa techniques, using the techniques of modern acupuncture is sufficient. Note, however, that the modern extraordinary vessel treatment styles generally use shallow insertions. Barely insert the needles; it is not necessary to "get the qi," particularly not the "dull, heavy, aching, distended" sensation associated with some modern methods of standing insertion. Since some practitioners feel that the technique employed is able to change the effect of the point needled, it is worthwhile to consider this aspect of treatment carefully. Successful modern practitioners use shallower insertion methods; it is worth considering that the classical practitioners also may have found a less assertive technique more successful.

Finally, there are passages in both the *Da Cheng* and *Ju Ying* where the problem itself is unclear. Remember that in the history of medicine diseases that no longer exist, or that are much less common, often appear. In this circumstance we have rendered the disease as a series of symptoms that describe the problem. Where possible we have tried to give some clear western disease names.

Ren Mai Symptomology

The *Nan Jing* symptom sets are based on the discussion found in the *Su Wen*. The author of the *Nan Jing* describes the following symptoms as indicative of problems associated with the ren mai:

> *Suffering or uncomfortableness of the insides, like a knot {a palpable lump}. Men can have seven kinds of lower warmer pain. Women can have lumps, or something collected or gathered in the lower abdomen.*[9]

The seven kinds of pain in men range from hernia to abdominal pain. Lumps in women come from a variety of sources, including congealed or stagnant blood. Wang Shu He expands the *Nan Jing* symptoms, describing eight types of lumps:

1. Shrimp lump
2. Blue lump
3. Abdominal lump
4. Yellow lump
5. Dry lump
6. Blood lump
7. Single lump
8. Turtle lump[10]

The shrimp lump seems to be named for its shape. The blue lump may be seen as a superficial blood vessel. Wang Shu He does not explain if the abdominal lump covers part of the abdomen or is inclusive of the whole abdomen. A yellow lump might reference a general yellow pallor in a specific area. The dry lump could relate to dry stools or constipation. The blood lump seems easily related to congealed blood. A single lump may be a differentiation from the other lumps, which could occur in multiples. The turtle lump, like the shrimp lump, would be most easily associated with a particular shape. A "congealed or coalesced" lump indicates an obstruction where something collects. It will move and have an irregular or changing shape.

The seven kinds of men's pain are:

1. Rebellious pain
2. Flat and round pain
3. Cold pain
4. Lump pain
5. Fu [府] pain
6. Pain that is accompanied by a palpitation or pulsing
7. Qi pain

Rebellious pain may be related to rebellious qi. Flat and round pain is less clear, possibly a description of the type of abdomen. Cold pain would be caused by or accompanied by cold and pain related to inflammation or swelling, as with a hernia. Fu pain may be associated with either a pulling or stretching pain or with pain in the lymph nodes. Pain accompanied by palpitation or pulsing seems straightforward; and qi pain would be most easily associated with stagnant qi. Wang Shu He also tells us that the character for ren [任] means pregnancy, and thus implies that it is the source of "life's nourishment." He argues that the use of this character means that the ren mai may be used for internal heart pain.[11]

It is hard to find a clear definition of these symptoms. Wang Shu He and the *Nan Jing* associate the ren mai with abdominal lumps in women, and sexual organ pain in men. Since lumps are often found in the abdomen upon palpation, knowledge of their significance is important. However, the descriptions are sufficiently vague to require further confirmation before we may assume that treatment of the ren mai is necessary. When we find a lump on palpation, we should investigate the ren mai to see if it is the appropriate treatment target.[12]

Wang Shu He indicates in the *Mai Jing* that when the ren mai is affected, one will feel something "like a ball at the horizontal side of the pulse {along the edges}." Symptoms will be: suffering from a feeling of wind in the abdomen, a feeling in the heart as if a stick were poking up from the lower abdomen, inability to lay down, and a feeling of tension. If the pulse is tight, thin, full and long, this too is a ren mai pulse. Symptoms will be: pain in the lower abdomen caused by movement, a sensation below the navel of pulling down to the pubic bone, stabbing pain in the sexual organs. Wang Shu He recommends treating three divisions below the navel (CV-4).[13]

Zhen Jiu Ju Ying — Ren Mai Treatments

Treat LU-7 then KI-6 for:

- cold pain and diarrhea: spleen
- post partum blood lump with pain or retention of normal post partum discharge (lochia): liver
- swollen and painful throat (pharyngitis or tonsillitis): stomach
- fetus dies and will not deliver: liver
- teeth swollen and painful: stomach, large intestine
- small intestine spasm pain (such as a hernia that protrudes on the abdomen): small intestine
- stagnation on one side of the abdomen with pain: liver, lungs
- vomiting saliva with pus and blood: lungs
- coughing with cold mucus: lungs
- pulling qi pain in the muscles below the ribs (or severe muscle tension between the scapulae or severe

tension at the side of the navel caused by cold wind invading the uterus): stomach

- stagnant food and digestive problems: stomach
- sharp pain of the umbilicus and abdomen: spleen
- pain of the heart and abdomen: spleen
- borborygmus and diarrhea: large intestine
- itchy, painful, bleeding hemorrhoids: large intestine
- heart pain and diarrhea associated with high fever (a shanghan symptom): spleen
- lumbar pain following labor: kidney, liver
- madness after labor: heart
- inability to speak after labor: pericardium
- inability to digest rice and grains: spleen
- stagnation on one side of the abdomen caused by alcohol, the food cannot pass: stomach, liver
- swelling, pain or abscess on the sides of the breast (mastitis): stomach
- stagnant blood lump in women: liver, kidney
- chronic external febrile disease (a shanghan symptom): gallbladder
- ceaseless vomiting: spleen, stomach
- blood in the urine: small intestine
- inability to pass urine: bladder
- constipation: large intestine
- bloody faeces: large intestine
- painful disease of the stomach/intestine: heart, stomach
- any lump: heart, stomach[14]

Chronic external febrile disease originates with a cold invasion and injury during the winter, then transforms to heat with the symptoms first appearing in the spring.

Zhen Jiu Da Cheng — Ren Mai Treatments

The *Zhen Jiu Da Cheng* indications for the ren mai are clear. The symptoms and diseases to be treated through the ren mai were presented as those treated by the master point—coupled point combination, LU-7 and KI-6. This is true for each of the extraordinary vessels. Since the indications are given as lists, rather than as text, we have quoted the context, but not the original format; that is, we have rearranged the translation in a more modern style for the readers' convenience. Symptoms that were grouped in the text are grouped in the list; these groupings indicate compound conditions. The diseases in the resulting list are in the order of the original text; however, there is no textual justification for assuming an identical order of importance or precedence.

LU-7 can mainly treat problems of the heart, abdomen, sides of the rib cage, diseases of the five yin organs. LU-7 and KI-6 together can treat:

- hemorrhoids
- nue, [瘧]
- swollen stools {enlarged stools}, with diarrhea
- drops of blood in the sputum
- hematuria and cough with mucus
- toothache, specially of the canine teeth, with swollen throat and difficulty urinating
- heart, chest and abdominal pain; when eating or drinking, it is hard to swallow and one sometimes chokes on the food
- after labor, the body becomes tight and rigid and the woman cannot speak
- lumbago
- blood problems with cold umbilicus
- miscarriage with retention of part of the afterbirth inside the uterus, the dead tissues causing cold to stagnate in the diaphragm (middle warmer)
- LU-7 can disperse an abscess of the breast.[15]

The term "nue" requires some explanation. Nue is usually translated as malaria, the "hot and cold" disease, but it does not necessarily refer only to malaria. However, the term does include malaria within the category of disease that it describes. Nue disease was first discussed in the *Su Wen*.[16] Research of nue disease shows that it is a general category, much like rebellious qi. Generally, nue is said to occur in the summertime, when the body is damaged by heat, and to manifest in the fall.[17] A disease of external invasion where "evil qi" is combated by the "correct qi," nue occurs when the external qi predominates.[18] It is associated with a damp wind attacking in the fall and the damp heat that triggers the attack.[19] People who suffer from nue, which can become chronic, tend to be susceptible to seasonal changes.[20] The disease is labelled hot nue, cold nue or simple nue according to whether heat manifests first, followed by chills, or chills followed by heat, or heat alone.[21] The seven emotions may also play a role, as do problems of the spleen and stomach, especially if there is mucus in the stomach.[22] The evil qi usually attacks the stomach meridian first.[23]

The major symptoms of nue are yawning followed by fear of cold and chills with shaking. The back and spine become painful. When the cold goes inside and the outside of the body becomes hot, the person will develop a splitting headache with thirst and an urge to drink cold drinks. The pulse will be generally wiry.[24] There are two common abdominal patterns. In the first pattern, there will be stagnation on the right side, usually relating to a deficient middle warmer. In the second pattern the skin of the abdomen will be tense and there will be a pulsing, lump or pressure pain on the stomach meridians.[25] According to the *Su Wen,*[26] and most authors,[27] if the disease recurs every day, it is easier to cure. If it recurs every two or three days, it is more difficult to cure. When it recurs daily it is still superficial, only in the meridians. When it recurs every two or three days, it is deeper, in the organs.[28] If the disease becomes chronic, the body may become weak.[29]

The *Zhen Jiu Da Cheng* mentions the ren mai, yin wei mai and the chong mai for treatment of nue disease. The emphasis in on the chong mai. There are also a variety of other treatments. The following is the advice of Waichi Sugiyama, a medical scholar of seventeenth century Japan:

> *For cold nue, one can first needle and then moxa: CV-12, LV-13, BL-20, BL-18, GV-14.*
>
> *A general treatment for nue disease is to select from and treat: GV-14, BL-13, BL-18, ST-25, GV-12, BL-40, LV-13, PC-5, SI-3, BL-57, BL-58, BL-60, KI-3, SP-4, BL-67, LI-4.*
>
> *If the disease is chronic in nature, apply moxa seventy times to BL-20.*[30]

These treatments may be used in conjunction with, or as a replacement for, the *Zhen Jiu Da Cheng* treatment of nue.

Zhen Jiu Da Cheng
Ren Mai Combination Treatments

The following treatments are combinations for the ren mai. The basic format, used for each of the extraordinary vessel points, is a symptom pattern followed by a list of recommended treatment points. The first point in the list is always the extraordinary vessel point featured, the remaining points are adjunctive. Since moxa is specified for certain points, we may assume that all the other points are needled. The order in which the points are treated seems important. Since the same point is occasionally treated twice in the same formula, we have assumed that the points are treated in sequence, not at once. Careful examination of these condition—point lists reveals the prototypes of what has become modern acupuncture. Note that the descriptions are compound symptom—condition statements related to point procedures. They require only the step of relating the condition to energetic states and the points to treatment qualities to become basic syndromes, which may be an indication of how an important and useful development in acupuncture evolved. These treatment combinations were thought of as treatments of both root and local problems.

Recommended points that are not located on the meridians have location descriptions given at the end of this chapter. Some of the treatments come from Dr. Yang, the author of the *Zhen Jiu Da Cheng*. This implies that the lists of treatments were compiled from other major sources. Some of the symptoms are unclear; we have translated these according to the *Jing Ming Zhong Yi Ci Dian, Concise Chinese Medical Dictionary*, the *Morohashi Encyclopedic Dictionary*, the *Zhen Jiu Xue, Acupuncture and Moxibustion Studies*, the *Shinkyu Byosho Gaku, Diseases and Configurations in the Study of Acupuncture and Moxibustion* and the advice of Dr. Chun Han Zhu, OMD, of the New England School of Acupuncture.

Ren mai treatment combinations are as follows:

- chronic bad smelling runny nose (rhinitis or sinusitis): LU-7 and BL-4, GV-23, GV-20, BL-12, LI-20
- nasal polyps or other growths in the nose that cause stagnation: LU-7 and yin tang, LI-20, GV-23, BL-12
- attack by wind, red face, high fever, headache: LU-7 and HT-5, LI-11, BL-60, LI-4

- attack by wind, susceptible to cold, coughing and panting: LU-7 and CV-17, BL-12, LI-4, GV-16
- attack by wind injures the four limbs, with fever, headache (like catching cold): LU-7 and LU-8, LI-11, LI-4, BL-54

In these cases, "attack by wind" refers to conditions that are like "catching cold." However, in other instances, the term refers more to conditions such as stroke, hemiplegia, and Bell's palsy. These latter symptoms could be internal conditions irritated by external wind or just internally generated wind.

- inside the abdomen is swollen and painful with diarrhea that will not stop: LU-7 and ST-44, ST-25, SP-6
- white or red diarrhea, the inside of the abdomen is cold with pain {possibly dysentery}: LU-7 and ST-28, CV-6, ST-26, ST-25, SP-6, ST-36
- front of the chest and both sides of the breast are red, swollen and painful: LU-7 and SI-1, PC-7, CV-17
- breast abscessed, swollen and painful, the baby is vomiting: LU-7 and LU-1, CV-17, SI-1, LV-1
- inside the abdomen is cold and painful with diarrhea that will not stop: LU-7 and ST-25, CV-12, CV-4, SP-6
- post partum blood stagnation with rebellious qi (with symptoms such as: dirty yellow face, lines on the nails, a palpable lump in the stomach, abdomen or ribcage area that does not move, constant pain, constipation or black stools): LU-7 and BL-18, BL-17, BL-23, SP-6
- coughing and panting with cold mucus and tight, contracting pain in the chest and diaphragm: LU-7 and BL-13, CV-17, ST-36
- chronic cough with blood and mucus in the saliva: LU-7 and BL-12, LU-9, CV-17
- panting and shortness of breath, mucus and qi stagnant in the chest: LU-7 and ST-40, KI-27, CV-17, ST-36

One tradition teaches that mucus originates in the "wrapping luo," the pericardium, the fatty fascial sac of the heart. The idea is that mucus begins "hidden in the pericardium." When the patient is diseased it follows the qi, rising up to the lungs, causing blockage and cough and finally manifesting as mucus. Mucus is seen as the unnecessary parts of the water system of the entire body; this relates it to triple warmer function.[31] Mucus diseases are said to be caused by internal heat, qi, wind pathologies, shock, fright, poor diet, alcohol, climatic heat, injury by cold, spleen or kidney deficient conditions. Mucus manifests chronically in alcoholics.

- loud raspy breathing, chest and diaphragm tight and painful: LU-7 and KI-26, CV-22, BL-13, ST-36
- loud panting, qi full, lungs feel swollen and the patient cannot lie down: LU-7 and KI-27, BL-12, LU-9, LU-1, ST-36, CV-17
- stuffed nose and cannot discern smells: LU-7 and LI-20, GV-23, BL-12
- runny nose (watery), skin feels rough, sneezing: LU-7 and GV-24, BL-13, LU-9, ST-36
- swelling of the neck in women (tuberculosis of the lymph nodes, red, swollen and painful), unable to lactate: LU-7 and SI-1, PC-7, CV-17, TW-1
- small pimple on the nipple {probably mastitis}: LU-7 and ST-18, SI-1, GB-21, CV-17
- stagnant pain inside the chest, unable to swallow: LU-7 and PC-7, PC-6, CV-17, ST-36
- five kinds of lumps in the neck {all some form of hyperthyroid condition, with palpitations, excitability, protruding eyes}, stone lump (hard), qi lump (soft like cotton), blood lump (stagnant blood or red with vascular spider), muscle lump, flesh lump (feels soft and empty on the interior): LU-7 and LI-18, SI-16, ST-12, KI-27, CV-17, LI-4, shi xuan (bleed), the extra point "above the throat" {perhaps a reactive point found on palpation above the larynx}.
- abscess or pimple in the mouth, halitosis (so bad that it is difficult to approach the patient): LU-7 and shi xuan, GV-26, jin jin, yu ye, CV-24, LI-4
- "absolute heat" in the triple warmer with abscess or pimple in the mouth: LU-7 and TW-1, TW-5, GV-26, LI-20, jin jin, yu ye, ST-4
- terrible halitosis: LU-7 and HT-9, HT-5, GV-26, shi xuan, jin jin, yu ye

- attack by heat with delirium, vomiting, almost comatose (severe sunstroke): LU-7 and BL-54, bai lao, GV-14, CV-12, LU-11, shi xuan, ST-36, LI-4
- attack by heat and difficulty urinating (mild sunstroke): LU-7 and KI-10, bai lao, CV-12, BL-54, CV-6, SP-9
- arms and legs contracting and spasming in children (childhood epilepsy): LU-7 and yin tang, GV-20, GV-26, PC-9, LV-1, LV-3, LI-4
- chronic "spleen wind" in children, eyes open and fixed, arms and legs spasming, bubbling saliva {like meningitis}: LU-7 and LV-1, BL-20, GV-20, GV-23, GV-26
- exhausted spleen, exhausted middle, exhausted kidneys: LU-7 and GV-26, SP-4, BL-20, CV-12, TW-1, KI-6
- black "sha" (infectious heat disease with black or dark red spots or pimples), abdominal pain, headache, fever, chills, tension pain of the lumbar or back areas, unable to sleep or lay down: LU-7 and bai lao, LU-3, BL-54, shi xuan
- white "sha" (infectious heat disease with white spots or pimples), abdominal pain, vomiting or diarrhea, four limbs cold, the fingernails are black, unable to sleep or lay down: LU-7 and PC-7, bai lao, LV-1, shi xuan
- black and white "sha," headache, thirst, large intestine diarrhea, chills, four limbs cold, borborygmus: LU-7 and BL-54, CV-17, GV-20, the area around CV-6, LV-1, GB-44, shi xuan[32]

The three conditions, "exhausted spleen," "exhausted middle" and "exhausted kidneys," are each a form of diabetes. In the earlier literature, diabetes was related to "exhaustion caused by thirst." Deficiency of the fluids, the jin and ye of the lungs, spleen or kidneys, caused fire-heat to increase. This, in turn, caused dryness and great thirst. In the *Su Wen* it is said that the following are the three "exhausted symptoms":

Stomach organ deficiency (eating much but still hungry),
Kidney thirst (drinking "100 cups" and still thirsty),
Mind and sexual desire unconnected or disharmonious.

KI-3 can be added to the treatment to ameliorate the disharmony of the mind and sexual desire, ST-36 to treat the hunger.

According to the *Su Wen* dryness of the earth element is the cause of the excessive thirst. Earth can not control the alchemical transformation of food and fluids. The term "exhausted middle" refers to heat in the middle warmer causing spleen deficiency. This "hidden yang" steams the stomach, exhausting the grain qi. One then becomes constantly hungry, able to eat twice as much, but unable to put flesh on the body. This is often accompanied by frequent urination. The term "exhausted kidney" refers to heat hidden in the lower warmer causing kidney deficiency with symptoms of thinness of the thighs and knees, sore joints, spermatorrhea, large consumption of fluids and therefore frequent urination having an unclear appearance. This is lower warmer diabetes.

Dr. Yang's Ren Mai Treatments

- reckless (spontaneous) bleeding and dizziness caused by blood problems: LU-7 and GV-26
- stagnant knot between the chest and diaphragm: LU-7 and KI-1, LU-11, CV-17, PC-6
- umbilical and abdominal pain: LU-7 and CV-17, PC-7, LU-1, SI-1, LU-9, SP-6
- inside the heart feels anxious, pressured or uncomfortable: LU-7 and SP-9, PC-6
- sound like insects in the ear {tinnitus}: LU-7 and HT-9, GB-2, PC-9, LI-1
- runny nose, dirty turbid mucus: LU-7 and GV-23, PC-6, LU-7 {again}, LI-11, LI-4
- shanghan with fever: LU-7 and BL-4, PC-6, LU-7 {again}, LU-8, LI-4[33]

The term "shanghan," injury by cold, refers to external invasion disease. Cold injures the body during the winter; the cold transforms to heat and symptoms begin to manifest. One can distinguish injury by cold from injury by wind through the absence of sweat in the former and presence of sweat in the latter.

Chong Mai Symptomology

In the "Four Ocean" chapter of the *Ling Shu*, upper and lower transportation points are described for the chong mai, which is seen as the ocean of the twelve meridians and the ocean of the blood. These points are BL-11, ST-37 and ST-38.[34] It is not clear whether these are trajectory, special or treatment points. Symptoms associated with these points denote a feeling of fullness in the body, for an excess blood condition; and a feeling of smallness in the body, for a deficient blood condition.[35]

The chong mai was clearly seen to relate to the blood. The association of the chong mai with ST-37 and ST-38, points that have strong effects on the digestive system, helps explain why one modern practitioner uses the chong mai to treat stomach ulcers.[36] The *Ling Shu* has another interesting discussion of the chong mai and its relationship to the blood and qi:

> *If the qi and blood are sufficient, the skin becomes healthy and the flesh has heat. If only the blood is sufficient, the blood moistens the skin and makes the body hair. Prenatally, women have sufficient qi, but not enough blood. The ren mai and chong mai cannot nourish the mouth and lips sufficiently, which is why women do not have moustaches or beards. In the eunuch, having the zong muscle {penis and testicles} cut off damages the chong mai. The beard and moustache do not grow because the chong mai cannot nourish around the mouth.*[37]

This passage relates the chong mai to what we now call hormonal function. We have seen potential relationships of the extraordinary vessels to the endocrine system in an earlier chapter.

The *Nan Jing* symptoms are clear:

> *When the chong mai has problems, the symptoms will be rebellious qi and tension or contraction of the lining.*[38]

Tension or contraction of the lining is tension of the abdomen and abdominal muscles. Wang Shu He explains these symptoms:

> *If the kidney qi is deficient, this deficiency damages the chong mai. The chong mai has rebellious qi, which does*

not rise up, making the lining tense with abdominal swelling and pain.[39]

This clarifies the *Nan Jing* symptoms. Other authors, Li Shi Zhen and Gao Wu, for example, concur that this is a reference to abdominal tension.[40]

According to Wang Shu He, it is a yang pulse if both pulses are floating. If both are sinking, it is a yin pulse. If both the yin and yang are full, this is a pulse of both the du and chong mai:

Radial Artery Pulse Cross-Sections

The pulse is felt both superficially and deep:

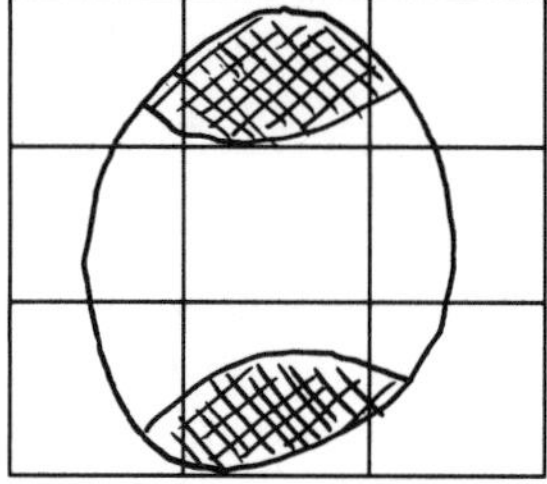

The pulse feels like two separate pulses:

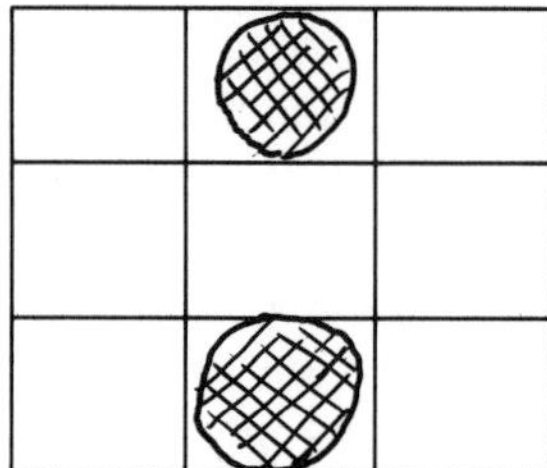

Figure 19

The chong mai and du mai combined are the way of the twelve meridians. If the chong and du mai do not function correctly, the twelve meridians will not return to the great meeting of the vessels (at LU-9). The patient will be in a trance, mad or idiotic. If the patient does not show these symptoms, the pulse diagnosis cannot possibly be correct.[41] In a chong mai pulse, the first and third positions will evidence the prison quality: deep, strong and hard. The pulse will rise and fall perpendicularly, and the symptoms will include a feeling of something in the chest that causes coldness or pain. If the middle pulse feels fuller and harder than the other positions, this too is a chong mai pulse. Symptoms will be: pain in the lower abdomen, pain caused by movement, the feeling that there is a stick pressing the heart, lumps, inability to become pregnant, dripping urine with incontinence, discomfort or fullness below the ribs {similar to chest distress}.[42]

The relationship of the kidney qi and the chong mai is also interesting, supporting the interpretation of a connection between the chong mai and the moving qi between the kidneys. This is explicitly stated in the *Tai Su* and implied by other texts. Li Shi Zhen, citing the *Ling Shu*, says:

> *When treating rebellious qi that rises to the upper parts, treat the places on the chest that are depressed {CV-17 or CV-22}. Below this, find a moving pulse and needle it. . . . . . For abdominal pain, which is related to the chong mai, put needles on the right and left moving pulses near the umbilicus. If this does not eliminate the pain immediately, treat qichong {ST-30}.*[43]

Gao Wu tells us that if there is rebellious qi and tension of the abdomen, choose points from KI-11 to KI-21.[44] We may infer that Gao Wu is referring to palpation of the points to find reaction, or examining the effects of each of the points to see if they treat the patient's symptoms.

Zhen Jiu Ju Ying — Chong Mai Treatments

SP-4, chong mai, meets at the heart and chest. Treat SP-4, then PC-6 for:

- nine kinds of heart pain: heart, stomach
- stagnant mucus, drooling and anguished: heart, chest
- umbilicus and abdomen swollen and painful: triple warmer, stomach
- pain at the side of the rib cage: heart, spleen
- following labor, loss of blood and spontaneous bleeding: master of the heart
- stagnant qi, food doesn't move: small intestine, stomach
- diarrhea that will not stop: large intestine, stomach
- pulling qi pain in the muscles below the ribs (or severe muscle tension between the scapulae or severe tension at the side of the navel caused by cold wind invading the uterus): heart, stomach
- the anus is painful following a heavy bout of diarrhea: large intestine
- a shanghan knot in the chest (evil qi is knotted in the chest, when the knot appears it causes pain below the

sternum that is tight on palpation): small intestine, heart
- stagnant water, alcohol mucus: liver, stomach
- full condition and discomfort in the abdomen, stomach disturbed, nausea and vomiting: stomach
- abdomen and sides swollen, full and painful: spleen, stomach
- wind in the intestines (blood in the stool caused by general weakness of the yin and yang organs and qi and blood disharmonies): large intestine, master of the heart
- anal prolapse: large intestine, lung
- stagnant qi (choking, rebellious full condition in the chest, belching that smells bad): heart, lungs
- stagnant food, food and fluids will not pass, constipation: stomach, spleen
- food lump (imbalance between the spleen and stomach, the area around CV-12 is full and painful and the patient will not like being touched at that point, there will be constipation and acid regurgitation), with pain: stomach, spleen
- in one side of the abdomen there is something that disturbs the digestive system hidden in the rib cage: small intestine, master of the heart
- postpartum lower abdominal pain caused by stagnant blood: small intestine, triple warmer
- problem on one side below the ribs caused by alcohol: stomach, triple warmer
- borborygmus: small intestine, stomach
- blood stabbing pain (sharp pain caused by blood stagnation): liver, spleen
- in children the spleen is dispersed (by heat) with symptoms of hidden heat in the spleen and stomach, heat in the flesh, dry mouth, lips dry, mouth sores, bad breath, thirst: spleen, kidney
- diarrhea with abdominal pain: large intestine, stomach
- stabbing pain in the chest: heart
- nue and heart pain: pericardium[45]

The term "knot in the chest" refers to a feeling of fullness and pain below the sternum. If this symptom is reported by the patient and on palpation the area is hard, with hardness extending down to the navel, and is uncomfortable when touched, this is a large knot in the chest. However, if it is only found on palpation, it is a small knot in the chest.

Zhen Jiu Da Cheng — Chong Mai Treatments

The *Zhen Jiu Da Cheng* gives the following list of symptoms for the chong mai:

SP-4 and PC-6 together can treat and balance the heart, abdomen, the five yin organs and:

- nine kinds of heart pain
- fullness in the chest or pressure in the heart with diaphragm problems (caused by spleen deficient mucus or damp spleen)
- evil qi knotted in the chest, causing pain below the heart (or sternum), with the urge to vomit, and vomiting after eating
- acute stomach upset (spasming or pain)
- too much alcohol or bad diet that causes lump formation (both yin and yang lumps)
- borborygmus
- water, food, qi diseases (improper fluid, food or air intake) causing diaphragm problems {belching, discomfort in the stomach — middle warmer problems}
- pain in the umbilicus
- sudden abdominal pain
- sides of the body swollen
- afterbirth, or parts thereof, retained following labor (causing coma or mental disease)
- watery diarrhea
- intestinal wind with nue and heart pain[46]

Intestinal wind may be either bleeding hemorrhoids or wind attacking the intestines damaging the blood and qi. The latter syndrome is evidenced by bleeding, diarrhea or bright colored blood that precedes the stools.

Zhen Jiu Da Cheng
Chong Mai Treatment Combinations:

- nine kinds of heart pain and the patient feels cold: SP-4 and PC-7, CV-12, SP-1
- fullness in the chest or pressure in the heart with diaphragm problems (caused by spleen deficient mucus or damp spleen), with deep pain in the chest: SP-4 and PC-8, CV-17, PC-5
- stagnation in the esophagus (rebellious full condition) with bad smelling belches, halitosis and an inability to swallow food and fluid {possibly cancer of the esophagus}: SP-4 and CV-17, ST-36, SP-3
- distended abdomen and umbilicus with undigested food: SP-4 and ST-25, CV-9, ST-44
- chronic pain in the sides or below the ribcage: SP-4 and TW-6, LV-13, GB-34
- watery diarrhea that will not stop, with tension and pain in the anus: SP-4 and CV-10, ST-25, KI-6
- deep {non palpable} stabbing pain in the chest: SP-4 and PC-6, PC-7, KI-26
- the sides of the ribcage are swollen and painful: SP-4 and GB-39, LV-13, GB-34
- distension and discomfort in the middle {warmer} with upset stomach and vomiting food {gastritis}: SP-4 and CV-12, SP-3, zhong kuei
- mucus in the stomach, vomiting clear water: SP-4 and CV-14, CV-12, ST-45
- food stagnant in the stomach with stabbing pain: SP-4 and CV-12, ST-36, ST-41
- nausea and vomiting, fullness in the chest or pressure in the heart with diaphragm problems (caused by deficient spleen mucus or damp spleen) and dizziness: SP-4 and CV-17, zhong kuei, ST-40
- nue of the heart causing physical and emotional overexcitement {such as angina and palpitations}: SP-4 and HT-7, BL-15, bai lao
- nue of the spleen causing dread of cold and abdominal pain: SP-4 and SP-5, BL-20, ST-36
- nue of the liver causing pale blue color, chills and high fever: SP-4 and LV-4, BL-18, GB-39

- nue of the lungs causing the heart to be cold and fearful, easily shocked or surprised (related to stress): SP-4 and LU-7, BL-13 , LI-4
- nue of the kidneys {with symptoms like} the overheating that results from alcohol consumption, causing the urge to drink much, and tension and pain of the spine and back: SP-4 and KI-4, BL-62, BL-23
- nue with high fever that is difficult to eliminate: SP-4 and PC-5, bai lao, GB-39
- nue with first cold then fever: SP-4 and SP-3, LI-11, PC-8
- nue with first fever then cold: SP-4 and LI-11, bai lao, GB-39
- nue with heart, chest pain: SP-4 and PC-6, CV-13, PC-7
- nue with headache, dizziness and vomiting mucus: SP-4 and LI-4, CV-12, LU-7
- nue with soreness of the bones and joints: SP-4 and BL-37, bai lao, KI-2
- nue with thirst (dry mouth included): SP-4 and TW-1, GV-26, PC-5
- nue of the stomach, always hungry but cannot eat: SP-4 and ST-45, BL-21, SP-2
- nue of the gallbladder with chills, fearfulness, nervous sensitivity, easily surprised, feeling of anxiousness when the patient lays down or sleeps: SP-4 and GB-41, BL-19, LV-14
- jaundice, four limbs swollen, profuse sweating (clothes wet): SP-4 and GV-9, bai lao, SI-4, CV-12, ST-36
- jaundice, one side of the body more colored than the other, skin, eyes and urine yellow: SP-4 and BL-20, SP-1, bai lao, GV-9, ST-36, SI-3
- grain jaundice, stagnant food causes "heart dizziness" {disturbs the heart}, the patient is mentally trying to reject or suppress some melancholic feelings {depression}, part of the body becomes yellower: SP-4 and BL-21, ST-44, GV-9, ST-36, SI-4, KI-10
- alcohol jaundice, both body and eyes yellow, deep heart pains, red spots on the face, yellow urine: SP-4 and BL-19, GV-9, BL-54, SI-3

- "weak jaundice," (weakness that only occurs in men from too much sex or poor lifestyle), body and eyes yellow, fever and chills, scanty urine: SP-4 and CV-4, BL-23, GV-9, KI-2[47]

There are said to be five kinds of the "yellow disease," jaundice. Each is caused by damp heat invading the middle warmer, spleen and stomach. Jaundice with yellow discoloration over one side of the body, the skin, eyes and urine, is associated with acute high fever. The heat stagnates in the stomach. The patient has a good appetite and sleeps well, but is tired when moving. "Grain jaundice" originally comes from overeating injuring the middle warmer, causing deficient stomach qi. Then, damp heat becomes excess creating dizziness, weird feelings in the heart and whole body discomfort. "Alcohol jaundice" arises from alcohol consumption and may be accompanied by dry nostrils and feverish legs. "Weak jaundice" is known as "male jaundice." The body looks overfatigued, usually related to too much sex, and there are fever and chills. This may be accompanied by fullness below the navel. There may be scanty urine that is difficult to pass.

Dr. Yang's Chong Mai Treatments

- irregular menses: SP-4 and CV-4, CV-6, ST-25, SP-6
- fullness and pain inside the chest: SP-4 and PC-8, HT-5, PC-7, CV-17
- mucus heat with a knot inside the chest: SP-4 and LU-7, PC-7, KI-1
- wind pain of the four limbs: SP-4 and LI-11, TW-5, GB-34, SP-6, LI-10, GB-31
- feeling of stagnation in the throat: SP-4 and LU-11, GB-20, KI-6, ST-6[48]

Du Mai Symptomology

Many commentators have offered treatment points for the du mai. The *Jinkui Yaolue Fanglun* of approximately 200 AD says, "For diseases of the du mai, put moxa on dazhui {GV-14} and taodao

{GV-13}."[49] In the *Su Wen*, in the same chapter that speaks of the trajectory of the du mai, it says:

> *Rebellious qi comes up from the small hara causing heart pain, with inability to pass urine or faeces. Women have an inability to become pregnant, protruding hemorrhoids, incontinence of urine and a dry throat. To treat these symptoms, treat a point on the bone {spine}. If the symptoms are terrible, treat the lower hara.*[50]

Li Shi Zhen explains that the point on the bone might be CV-1 and the point on the hara might be CV-7.[51]

The *Nan Jing* tells us, "The spine is tight and rebellious."[52] Wang Shu He explains this by giving a treatment for these symptoms:

> *If the du mai is attacked by evil, the spine will become tight and rebellious; treat with moxa on shenzhu {GV-12}.*[53]

Some commentators translate "tightness and rebelliousness" as epilepsy;[54] however, it may be simply rigidity of the spine or back muscles.

The du mai pulse is a pulse where the first and third positions are floating, yet rise and fall "perpendicularly" {suddenly}, with symptoms of lumbar and back pulling pain with an inability to lay down. In adults, there will be epilepsy, in children, wind spasms. If the middle pulse is floating with sudden pain in the upper and lower parts of the body, this too is a du mai pulse. Symptoms will be movement causing pain, coldness of the lumbar, back and knees. In adults there will be epilepsy, in children wind spasms. Wang Shu He recommends treating these last two symptoms with moxa on the "top of the head."[55]

Zhen Jiu Ju Ying — Du Mai Treatments

Treat SI-3 then BL-62 for:

- tension and spasms of the arms and legs: liver
- shaking of the arms and legs: liver, triple warmer
- head wind pain: triple warmer, bladder
- chronic shanghan: bladder

- profuse night sweating: lung, heart
- attacked by wind {stroke}, unable to speak: liver meridian
- toothache: stomach, large intestine
- epilepsy, vomiting bubbly saliva: stomach
- tension and pain of the lumbar and back: kidney
- pain in the muscles or tendons and bones: liver, stomach
- stagnant throat: kidney, lung, stomach
- swelling and pain of the cheek and chin: stomach, small intestine
- shanghan, injury by cold causing pain or stiffness of the back of the neck: bladder
- swelling and pain of the knees and shin: kidney
- numbness of the arms and legs: stomach
- swollen and red eyes: liver, heart
- headache from shanghan, injury by cold: bladder
- inability to sweat: lung, stomach
- wind makes the eyes tear: liver, gallbladder
- tetanus: liver
- post partum spontaneous sweating with dread of wind: lung
- throat spasms: lung, liver
- pain in the shin, knee and thigh: stomach
- bi {numbness and spasming} of the hands: large intestine[56]

Zhen Jiu Da Cheng — Du Mai Treatments

The *Zhen Jiu Da Cheng* tells us that SI-3 controls diseases of the head, face, neck and back of the neck, and that SI-3 and BL-62 together will treat:

- Spasms, contractions or shaking of the arms and legs
- external wind
- external wind as in epilepsy, with inability to speak after falling down
- epilepsy
- headaches with eyes swollen and tearing
- pain from the knee or thigh areas that radiates to the lumbar or back areas

- neck tension on one side
- shanghan
- teeth (gums) and throat swollen (including mumps)
- arms and legs numb
- tetanus
- night sweating[57]

One tradition teaches that epilepsy begins if a pregnant mother receives a shock or fright such that the shen in the baby's heart is disturbed, inducing a prenatal epileptic condition. This form of epilepsy is said to be hard to treat. Forms of epilepsy brought on by postnatal trauma would be easier to treat.

Zhen Jiu Da Cheng — Du Mai Treatment Combinations

- tightness and spasming of the arms and legs, difficulty stretching: SI-3 and ST-36, LI-11, LV-2, GB-34
- no strength of the arms and legs, unable to walk, difficulty grasping: SI-3 and LI-4, LI-11, SI-4, LV-3, GB-39, SP-4, GB-34
- tension, pain and immobility of the neck and nape of the neck: SI-3 and CV-24, GB-20, GV-16
- redness and swelling of the glands on and under the cheeks and jaws {possibly including mumps}: SI-3 and ST-5, ST-6, LI-4
- feeling of something stuck in the throat, inability to swallow even a drop of water: SI-3 and CV-22, LI-1, KI-6, shi xuan
- tonsillitis that affects both tonsils: SI-3 and LU-11, jin jin, yu ye, shi xuan
- tonsillitis that affects one tonsil: SI-3 and TW-1, CV-22, LI-4
- unilateral or bilateral "head wind" with pain along the edges of the forehead: SI-3 and LU-7, LI-4, the visible blood vessel around tai yang, GB-5, TW-23
- pain at the lateral ends of the eyebrows: SI-3 and BL-2, GB-14, yin tang, LI-4, ST-8
- head and eyes dizzy, with pain on tai yang: SI-3 and LI-4, the visible blood vessel around tai yang, ST-8

- tightness of the head and neck with a feeling of having the head pulled backwards towards the shoulders: SI-3 and CV-24, GV-20, GB-21, TW-3
- dizziness and headache from alcohol consumption {hangover}, inability to listen to others: SI-3 and KI-1, LU-7, bai lao, LI-4
- eyes red and swollen with tearing that will not stop in a strong wind: SI-3 and BL-2, LI-4, xiao gukong, GB-41
- infection that leads to septicemia or tetanus, high fever and tension: SI-3 and LV-1, LI-4, LV-2, shi xuan, blood let from the visible blood vessel around tai yang[58]

A head wind is a deep, rather than a superficial, headache. It may be related to a susceptibility to wind evil that causes symptoms of headache, dizziness, or paralysis similar to Bell's palsy. This category may also be related to migraines.

Dr. Yang's Du Mai Treatments

- coughing, panting, cold mucus: SI-3 and LU-7, KI-1, BL-62, BL-13, CV-24, TW-23
- head and eyes feel dizzy: SI-3 and GB-20, GV-4, LI-4
- tension, hardness, tightness in the head and back of the neck: SI-3 and CV-24, GV-16, GB-20, LI-4
- toothache: SI-3 and LU-7, GV-26, ST-6, lu xi, LU-9, LI-4
- deafness, hardness of hearing: SI-3 and GB-2, LI-1, HT-9, PC-9
- tetanus: SI-3 and CV-24, LI-4, ba xie, SI-3 {again}, TW-5, the "four gates" {LV-3 and LI-4}[59]

Dai Mai Symptomology

When Wang Shu He describes the use of moxa on LV-13 as a method of treating dai mai disease,[60] he also lists the diseases that the *Nan Jing* describes as caused by dai mai imbalance:

Fullness and looseness of the abdomen, with a feeling of sitting in cold water.[61]

The "sitting in cold water" sensation may be literally interpreted; patients will describe the feeling as that of sitting in a tub with water up to the waist. Generally, it references pain and cold in the lumbar and sacral area.

In a dai mai problem, the pulse will feel as though it were "twisting" to the right and left with symptoms of umbilical, abdominal and lumbar pain or the feeling of something like a stick pressing against the groin.[62]

Quoting from the *Ming Tang Textbook*, Li Shi Zhen says that the symptoms of the dai mai are:

> *The lumbar and abdomen are like a balloon filled with water, there is a feeling of cold in the small abdomen with pain, tight anus, irregular menses and red or white discharge.*[63]

He continues by stating that these conditions can be treated by needling GB-26 to a depth of 0.6 divisions or applying moxa seven times.

Zhen Jiu Ju Ying — Dai Mai Treatments

Treat GB-41 then TW-5 for:

- swelling and pain on top of the foot: stomach
- numbness of the hands and feet: small intestine
- shaking of the hands and fingers: liver, master of the heart
- red eyes, cold tearing: bladder
- swollen and painful throat {pharyngitis or tonsillitis}: triple warmer
- tightness and spasming of the arms and legs: liver, kidney
- pain in the sides and ribs: gallbladder
- toothache: stomach, large intestine
- heat of the hands and feet: master of the heart
- shanghan with diarrhea: bladder

- inguinal joint pain: gallbladder
- leg and knee swollen: stomach, liver
- lack of control over the four limbs: gallbladder
- head wind {deeper chronic, recurrent headache or headache with dizziness, Bell's palsy, itchiness of the head with severe dandruff, swollen head}: bladder
- top of the head swollen: bladder
- itchiness and floating wind, {puffiness of the skin, as in allergic reactions}: lung
- body swollen: kidney, stomach
- body numbness: liver, spleen
- head and eye dizziness: bladder
- muscle spasms and bone pain: liver, stomach
- pain in the cheek and chin: large intestine
- thunder head wind: gallbladder
- eyes swollen and painful: liver, heart
- stroke {attack by wind}, cannot raise the arms and legs: kidney
- deafness: kidney, gallbladder[64]

Zhen Jiu Da Cheng — Dai Mai Treatments

The *Zhen Jiu Da Cheng* says that GB-41 mainly treats diseases of the four limbs. Using GB-41 and TW-5 together one can treat:

- Hemiplegia of the arms and legs, with inability to raise them {like stroke}
- pain, fever, numbness and spasms (anywhere in the body)
- head wind pain
- swelling from the back of the neck to the chin
- red and swollen eyes with vertigo
- toothache
- deafness
- swollen throat
- "floating wind" with itching and muscular tension {a skin rash or allergy}
- thigh pain and the sides of the body swollen, with an imbalance of one side of the body from the ribs down to the legs[65]

Zhen Jiu Da Cheng
Dai Mai Treatment Combinations

- chronic swelling and pain on the dorsum of the foot: GB-41 and LV-2, BL-62
- numbness of the arms and legs (difficulty feeling itchiness or pain in the limbs): GB-41 and LV-3, LI-11, PC-7, LI-4, ST-36, TW-3
- both legs shaking and difficulty walking: GB-41 and LV-3, BL-60, GB-34
- both hands shaking and inability to hold anything: GB-41 and PC-3, SI-4, LI-4, TW-3
- spasming, tightness and inability to open the toes: GB-41 and GB-40, SP-4, GB-34, wheat grain size moxa five times on top of the toes with toes bent (on the middle joints)
- fingers numb, pain when bending and straightening: GB-41 and LU-5, LI-5, TW-3, wu hu, wheat grain size moxa five times on the tops of the fingers with the hands clenched in a fist {on the middle joints}
- heat in the soles of the feet {damp heat}: GB-41 and KI-1, BL-64, LI-4
- external ankles red and swollen: GB-41 and BL-60, GB-40, KI-6
- feeling of heat on the dorsum of the feet with pain in the joints of the five toes: GB-41 and ST-42, GB-43, shi xuan
- heat in both hands with pain in the five fingers: GB-41 and TW-4, TW-2, LI-4
- both knees red, swollen and sore {"crane knee wind," related to gout}: GB-41 and LV-7, LV-2, GB-31, GB-34
- bone pain in the hands and arms: GB-41 and LU-9, SI-4, PC-7
- lumbar and groin pain {"sudden cold pain," a sharp stabbing pain, possibly hernia}: GB-41 and GB-27, BL-54, SP-6
- pain of the whole arm related to problems of the shoulder and back: GB-41 and GB-21, LI-11, TW-3
- thigh and bladder pain: GB-41 and GB-30, BL-54, GB-34

- gout pains: GB-41 and GB-21, ST-36, LI-11, BL-54, LI-4, LV-2, tian ying
- wind bi, moving pain in the four limbs {cold damp evil attacks the joints or meridians}: GB-41 and LI-11, BL-54, ST-36, tian ying:
- floating wind, whole body itching {itchy rashes, allergies}: GB-41 and GV-20, bai lao, GV-4, visible blood vessel around tai yang, LI-11, GB-31, GB-39, CV-9, CV-6, SP-10, BL-54
- redness, swelling, pain and tension on the head and back of the neck: GB-41 and CV-24, GB-20, GB-21, GV-16
- deficient kidney lumbar pain, difficulty moving, strained movements: GB-41 and BL-23, GV-6, BL-54
- lumbar pain from strain: GB-41 and GV-6, GV-2, BL-23, BL-54
- deficient, damp, stagnant lumbar pain, with no power of activity: GB-41 and GV-6, GV-2, BL-23, BL-54
- whole body weak, no energy in the four limbs: GB-41 and bai lao, BL-15, ST-36, CV-4, BL-38
- stabbing pain below the rib cage with a palpable lump {probably liver related}: GB-41 and LV-13, TW-6, CV-12, PC-7, GB-34[66]

Tian ying is an extra point that is similar to an "ah shi" point. Locate the painful point that is made comfortable or is relieved by pressure. Use a long needle with strong stimulation, then bleed the point.

Dr. Yang's Dai Mai Treatments

- spasming of the arms and legs: GB-41 and TW-3, LU-5, GB-39, ba xie, LI-5, GB-34
- wind bi of the four limbs: GB-41 and ST-36, BL-54, GV-4, tian ying, LI-11, TW-5
- pain in the knees and shins: GB-41 and LV-2, GB-39, LV-3, eyes of the knees, ST-36, GB-34
- cold bi pain of the thigh: GB-41 and the four gates (LV-3, LI-4), GB-39, GB-31, GB-30, SP-6

- cold bi pain of the arm: GB-41 and GB-21, LI-11, ST-36, TW-5
- all joints painful {sharp, almost burning pain, severe arthritis}: GB-41 and BL-42, GB-39, GV-4, TW-5[67]

Yin and Yang Qiao Mai Symptomology

In discussing a disease of the yang qiao mai and its treatment, the *Su Wen* explains exactly why BL-62 was chosen as the yang qiao starting and treatment point:

> *If evil visits the vessel of the yang qiao, the person has eye pain, which starts at the internal canthus of the eye. Insert the needle half a division below the lower part of the external malleolus. For the left, insert to the right; for the right, insert to the left. One hour later, the pain will be cured.*[68]

This treatment point has the same location as BL-62. The needling instructions are brief, though interesting, as we find one of the earliest references to an asymmetrical or topological treatment. The *Ling Shu* describes more symptoms of the yin and yang qiao mai with reference to the eyes:

> *If the qi of the yin qiao mai is excess, the eyes are closed and unable to open. If the qi of the yang qiao mai is excess, the eyes are opened and unable to close.*[69]

This may be related to a thyroid condition — for example, hyperthyroidism. A modern commentary, the *Nei Jing Jie Po Sheng Li Xue*, states that these symptoms are related to the tonus of the optic nerve.[70] The *Su Wen* and *Ling Shu* describe other symptoms related to the yin and yang qiao mai. When the *Su Wen* describes how to treat lumbar pain where the patient is unable to raise the legs while laying down, the instructions are to treat BL-61 or BL-62.[71] These points are in the same area that the *Su Wen* recommends for treatment of yang qiao symptoms. The *Ling Shu* describes a treatment for red eyes with pain around BL-1 by suggesting for treatment that we "choose a point" from the yin qiao mai trajectory.[72] Li Shi Zhen states that the point referenced is KI-8, the accumulation point of the yin qiao mai.[73]

The *Nan Jing* defines diseases of the yin and yang qiao mai in terms of the relative tension of the medial and lateral muscles of the legs above the malleoli.

> *In yang qiao mai disease, there is tightness of the yang side, and looseness of the yin side. In yin qiao mai disease, there is looseness of the yang side and tension of the yin side.*[74]

This was interpreted by Wang Shu He as tightness of the muscles above the external malleolus with a relative tension of the muscles above the internal malleolus, for the yang qiao mai. For the yin qiao mai, he indicates tightness of the muscles above the internal malleolus, with relative looseness above the external malleolus.[75] Interestingly, he also proposed treating KI-6 with moxa for hot diseases of the yin qiao mai. Often in modern practice, when hot conditions are found, moxa is contraindicated. This has not always been so. In modern Japanese practice the recommendation is to find a corresponding cold or cool condition elsewhere in the body and use moxa to treat the hot condition indirectly. For diseases of the yang qiao mai, he says:

> *If each of the yang meridians becomes full or excess, the excess energy goes to the yang qiao mai, which receives the evil, but the disease stays at the yang part of the extraordinary vessels. This is why the yin becomes loose, and the yang tense; this is the disease.*
> *If the yang disease is cold, treat GB-20.*[76]

If the pulses on both sides are floating (a yang pulse), thin and tiny, and if a yin pulse (deeper) is undetectable, this is a yin or yang qiao mai pulse. Accompanying symptoms will be: attraction to ghosts, demons and evil beings, "wind death," trance states. If a close relative dies, and the patient misses the deceased terribly (over-grieving), this too can bring another misfortune. Yang qiao disease is also indicated by tension or tightness as described in the *Nan Jing*.[77] The modern text, the *Nei Jing Jie Po Sheng Li Xue*, comments that this idea of relative tension and looseness of the muscles might be muscle spasms resulting from changes at the level of the spinal nerves.[78]

When Li Shi Zhen comments on diseases of the yin and yang qiao mai, his treatments are surprisingly similar to those of Wang Shu He:

For the yang qiao mai one will find symptoms of:

- wiriness of the anterior portions of the radial pulses
- lumbar or back pain
- epilepsy
- apoplexy
- crying like a sheep
- dread of cold
- hemiplegia
- numbness or tightness of the body (if the radial pulse is tiny and rough, this is wind epilepsy)

The treatment point for the yang qiao is GB-39, however if the yang disease is cold, needle GV-16 and GB-20.

For the yin qiao mai one can find symptoms of:

- wiriness of the posterior portions of the radial pulses
- epilepsy
- hot or cold symptoms
- numbness of the skin
- pain in the lower abdomen
- pulling pain from the lumbar and iliac crest areas to the sexual organs
- continuous discharge in women

Yin diseases are always hot, even if no heat is apparent. Moxa KI-6 and GB-34. For daytime epilepsy, moxa a point on the yang qiao mai. For nighttime epilepsy, moxa a point on the yin qiao mai.[79]

Zhen Jiu Ju Ying — Yin and Yang Qiao Mai Treatments

Treat BL-62 then SI-3 for:

- stiff and painful lumbar and back: bladder
- discomfort and pain of any or all joints: kidney, liver

- inability to raise arms and legs: stomach, lung
- shanghan, injury by cold with headache: bladder
- swelling and fullness of the whole body: stomach
- spontaneous sweating of the head and face: stomach
- epilepsy: liver
- red and swollen eyes: bladder
- attack by wind with spontaneous sweating {catching cold}: stomach
- head wind itching pain: gallbladder
- pain in the eyebrow bone (from sinusitis or rhinitis): bladder
- thunder head wind: gallbladder
- pain in the arms and hands: large intestine
- cold arms: triple warmer
- spontaneous sweating after labor: kidney
- epistaxis: lungs
- tetanus: liver
- swelling and pain of the joints: kidney, liver
- swelling and pain of the thighs and knees: stomach
- deafness: kidney
- numbness of the arms and legs: gallbladder
- breast pain or pain on breast feeding {possibly mastitis}: stomach
- head wind that follows washing the head: bladder
- spasms of the arms and legs: liver, kidney
- dread of wind after labor: kidney[80]

Treat KI-6 then LU-7 for:

- throat swollen and feels closed: stomach
- cold pain with urination: kidney, liver
- rough, dripping urination that won't pass: bladder
- blood dizziness in women: liver, kidney
- stagnant bladder qi with pain {possibly cystitis}: bladder
- retained afterbirth: liver
- pain of the umbilicus and abdomen: spleen
- small intestine swollen and full: small intestine
- bleeding from the wall of the intestine: large intestine
- food and fluids immediately vomited, "upside down" stomach: stomach

- alcoholism in males, lump on one side {cirrhosis or hepatitis} and stagnation of food: lungs, liver
- borborygmus, diarrhea, abdominal pain: large intestine
- feeling of fullness and discomfort in the abdomen: stomach
- undigested food {in the stools}: stomach
- following labor, stagnation of blood causes pain in the lower abdomen: stomach, liver
- difficult labor: kidney, liver
- watery diarrhea: spleen
- nausea and vomiting: stomach
- yin lump caused by alcohol {cirrhosis or hepatitis}: spleen
- pulling qi pain in the muscles below the ribs (or severe muscle tension between the scapulae, or severe tension at the side of the navel caused by cold wind invading the uterus): stomach
- qi lump {movable stagnant gas lump with dull pain in the intestines}: spleen, liver, kidney
- bi symptoms caused by alcohol: stomach, liver
- stagnant qi in the upper part of the middle warmer: master of the heart
- constipation: large intestine
- deficient spleen with food lump, stagnant food, skin becomes dirty yellow, face puffy, legs swollen, mouth bitter, legs sore, abdomen swollen, diarrhea: spleen, stomach
- hot feet: master of the heart[81]

Zhen Jiu Da Cheng *Yin and Yang Qiao Mai Treatments*

The *Zhen Jiu Da Cheng* gives the following sets of symptoms for the two pairs of points:

KI-6 mainly treats diseases of the yin and yang organs. KI-6 and LU-7 together can treat:

- the feeling of something stuck in the throat
- urinary incontinence, bladder qi pain

- borborygmus
- alcohol lump in the abdomen and around the umbilicus {cirrhosis or hepatitis}
- vomiting and diarrhea
- stomach is upside down {painful stomach} and hard stools {could be physically hard stools or difficulty passing stools}
- difficult labor causing coma or lumps
- wind in the intestines {bloody stools} and bleeding from the anus
- inside the diaphragm it feels comfortable and there is a feeling of plum pit qi in the throat {usually seen in hysteria}

BL-62 controls evil wind of the four limbs {paralysis}, abscess and poison diseases. BL-62 and SI-3 together can treat:

- dread of wind
- spontaneous sweating
- headache
- thunder head wind
- lumbar and back tight when bending, thighs swollen and tight
- red and painful eyes with soreness between the eyebrows
- arms and legs numb
- upper arm cold
- pre- or postpartum superficial, large breast abscess {mastitis caused by stagnant heat. Internally, during pregnancy the qi of the uterus becomes excess, causing stagnation and heat evil. Externally, after labor, heat stagnates in the breast causing abscess formation}.
- deafness
- epistaxis
- epilepsy
- joint pain
- sweating from the head
- one side of the body feels full and swollen[82]

Zhen Jiu Da Cheng
Yin Qiao Mai Treatment Combinations

- incontinence of urine or a feeling of stagnation; the urine drips but does not stream: KI-6 and SP-9, SP-6, TW-1, LI-4
- cold pain of the lower abdomen, voluminous urination: KI-6 and CV-6, CV-4, BL-23, SP-6
- seven kinds of strong, acute pain in the bladder, with "running piglet" {a lump related to the kidneys that causes a sensation of something rising}: KI-6 and LV-1, the area around CV-6, KI-1, SP-6, BL-20, PC-7, a point three divisions up from LV-8

These seven kinds of strong, acute pain of the bladder are often liver related. These may come one day before weather changes; the patient will be susceptible to the weather. Often, when palpating the abdomen, one will find tightness below the ribs (chest distress) or tightness to the side of the navel. On palpation the sensation radiates to the inguinal joint or into the testicles.

- swollen testicle {caused by mucus dampness, stagnant blood or liver heat}: KI-6 and LV-1, LV-8, KI-2, SP-6, ST-29, the point three divisions up from LV-8, BL-28, BL-23
- breast problem {where the breast develops raised lines that radiate out from the nipple} with acute pain in the lower abdomen or back {hernia related} that sometimes causes pain in heart: KI-6 and GB-26, KI-1, KI-3, LV-1
- incontinence of urine with blood in the urine and sexual organ pain {urinary infection}: KI-6 and KI-10, KI-1, SP-6
- spermatorrhea with white, unclear sperm and frequent urination: KI-6 and CV-4, BL-30, KI-3, SP-6
- dreams of sex with a {Chinese} demon, spermatorrhea: KI-6 and CV-3, BL-38, BL-15, KI-2, BL-23
- difficult labor, during and after labor the baby disturbs the mother's mind and spirit; retention of parts of the afterbirth: KI-6 and CV-14, LI-4, SP-6, BL-67 (moxa)

- women with constipation: KI-6 and BL-62, SP-9, SP-6, KI-3
- pain in the abdomen and umbilicus following labor, with constant discharge: KI-6 and CV-9, CV-4, BL-38, SP-6
- in women, spleen qi problems; blood worms, water worms, qi worms, stone worms:[83]
  TW-6, SP-6; KI-6 and CV-17, CV-9 for water worms;
  CV-4, CV-6, ST-36, LV-2 for blood worms;
  SP-4 for qi worms;
  ST-44 for stone worms
- "separated blood," "simple abdomen," "qi panting:" KI-6 and CV-10, CV-17, CV-6, ST-36, LV-2
- in women the blood and qi become weak, head and eyes dizzy: KI-6 and BL-23, GV-20, BL-38, LI-11, LI-4, GB-39
- in old people, weak energy, arms and legs hard to move, especially hard to lift: KI-6 and BL-57, GB-34, GB-41, KI-3, LU-5, LI-4
- delirium, vomiting or diarrhea, arms and legs cramping: KI-6 and BL-64, ST-36, BL-57, LI-11, SI-4, LU-5, GB-34
- cold damp beri-beri, fever with much pain: KI-6 and LV-3, BL-54, SP-6
- deficient kidney beri-beri, redness and swelling, high fever that will not pass: KI-6 and ST-30, KI-3, SP-4, SP-6, SP-10, BL-54
- dry beri-beri, patella, internal ankle, all fingers and/or toes painful: KI-6 and LV-7, BL-60, GB-39, BL-54, GB-34, SP-6
- whole body swollen, full and puffy {water}: KI-6 and CV-6, ST-36, LI-11, LI-4, ST-44, LV-2, SP-6
- heart and abdomen swollen and big: KI-6 and CV-12, CV-17, CV-9, SP-6
- the lower abdomen is swollen like a drum, "qi panting": KI-6 and CV-17, CV-6, CV-9, ST-36, LV-2, SP-6
- four limbs face and eyes swollen: KI-6 and GV-26, LI-4, ST-36, GB-41, LI-11, SP-6
- weakness in women, skinny body, red and white discharge: KI-6 and bai lao, BL-23, CV-4, SP-6
- chronic coldness of the uterus with sterility: KI-6 and ST-25, SP-6, the uterus point (three divisions lateral to CV-3)

- in women, the water meridians pass correctly, but they suffer from headache, dizziness, pain in the kidney and lower abdomen areas: KI-6 and GB-35, ST-44, LI-4
- uterus and monthly water imbalance {monthly distension or edema}, pain in the umbilicus or abdomen: KI-6 and BL-23, SP-6, CV-4
- difficult labor, baby does not deliver: KI-6 and LI-4, SP-6, du yin[84]

The reference to the mother's mind and spirit states that the child "squeezes, holds the mother's mind so that it cannot descend," describing a mother whose attention cannot leave the child and who is thus unable to relax.

The term "worm" refers to one of three problems:

1. Tapeworm that causes a lump formation injuring the liver and spleen; the luo vessels stagnate and protrude.
2. Heat and pain in the lower abdomen with white unclear urine.
3. Male sexual disease (more psychological than physical, such as excessive thoughts about sex).

"Separated blood" could refer to septicemia or blood poisoning. The symptoms are: very high fever, coma, delirium, vomiting blood, epistaxis, bloody stools. These may be related to problems of the heart, liver and kidney. The "simple abdomen" is a problem in the lower part of the abdomen. "Qi panting" is likely shortness of breath, dyspnea.

Dr. Yang's Yin Qiao Mai Treatments

- both qi and blood worms {any of the three worm symptoms described above}: KI-6 and LV-2, CV-4, CV-9, SP-4, CV-6, GB-41
- heat in the five hearts: KI-6 and PC-6, KI-1, shi xuan, PC-7, LI-4, BL-17, BL-19
- chest pain, feeling of qi pushing or pressing: KI-6 and HT-5, PC-7

- suffering with a feeling of pressure and uncomfortableness in the heart, stressed {suffers shock}: KI-6 and BL-15, PC-6, HT-7
- the esophagus and trachea feel stagnant like something is stuck: KI-6 and LU-11, GB-20, KI-6 (again)
- deficient yang, the patient is like a corpse: KI-6 and BL-15, KI-2, BL-23, CV-3, SP-6[85]

Zhen Jiu Da Cheng — Yang Qiao Mai Combination Treatments

- tension in the lumbar area, difficulty bending: BL-62 and GV-2, BL-38, BL-54
- joint pain, causing emotional distress, pulling pain in the lumbar part of the back: BL-62 and LI-14, LI-11, BL-60, GB-34
- after apoplexy, the patient has lost the power of concentration and the ability to disseminate and is comatose or semi comatose: BL-62 and PC-9, GV-20, LV-1, yin tang, LI-4
- inability to speak following apoplexy: BL-62 and LU-11, GV-21, GV-26, CV-17, LI-4, GV-15
- hemiplegia following apoplexy: BL-62 and LI-10, SI-4, LI-4, GB-39, LV-2, GB-31, SP-6
- one side of the body weak from an attack by wind, with pain that is not responsive to, or related to, seasonal, climatic or biorhythmic changes: BL-62 and GB-39, LU-9, LI-11. LI-15, ST-36, BL-60
- four limbs spasming following apoplexy: BL-62 and LI-12, LI-9, LU-10, GB-31, LV-7, SP-6
- hemiplegia, hand and leg weak, cannot hold or grasp: BL-62 and TW-13, SI-4, LI-4, LV-2, GB-31, GB-34
- hemiplegia of the face or spasming of one side of the face: BL-62 and LI-4, LU-9, shi xuan, GB-1, ST-6 (in this case ST-6 should be 0.1 divisions forward towards ST-4); disperse the points on the affected side or moxa the points fourteen times
- cramping of the body, eyes unfocussed following apoplexy: BL-62 and GV-20, bai lao, LI-4, LV-2, LI-11, shi xuan, GB-34

- mouth tight and unable to open, difficulty speaking following apoplexy: BL-62 and ST-4 (slightly towards ST-6), GV-26, LI-4
- pain in the lumbar spine, neck and back: BL-62 and BL-23, GV-26, GB-21, BL-54
- lumbar pain, hard to move the leg, hurts when moved: BL-62 and KI-2, BL-38, BL-54, BL-23
- poisoning on the dorsum of the foot (possibly abscess, infection or blood stagnation, purple, discolored area): BL-62 and ST-44, GB-43, LV-2, BL-54
- poisoning on the dorsum of the hand: BL-62 and TW-2, TW-3, LI-4, TW-5
- poisoning of the back of the hand and arm: BL-62 and LU-3, LI-11, BL-54[86]

Mr. Yang's Yang Qiao Mai Treatments

- abscess on the lumbar area: BL-62 and BL-54, GB-43, shi xuan, LI-11, TW-2, PC-6, TW-5
- pain on one side of the body: BL-62 and LU-9, ST-36, LI-11
- poisoning in the area of the hair from the front of the ear down to the chin: BL-62 and tai yang, BL-62 (again), KI-3, LI-4, TW-5
- deeply rooted abscess on the head: BL-62 and bai lao, LI-4, BL-62 (again), GV-18, BL-54
- headache, hard to bend down or over: BL-62 and BL-62 (again), BL-63, CV-24
- hard to move or twist the neck or nape of the neck: BL-62 and SI-3, LI-4, CV-24[87]

Yin and Yang Wei Mai Symptomology

The basic symptoms of the wei mai are noteworthy because they concern the emotional aspects of disease. The *Su Wen* indicates the following for the yang wei mai:

> *For swelling and pain on the lumbar area, or irritability and a swollen spot on the painful area, insert the needle*

> *into the vessel of the yang wei. The place {to treat} is on the external aspect of the leg, ten divisions above the bottom of the heel, where it meets tai yang.*[88]

This point is possibly GB-35.[89]

For the yin wei mai one might find these symptoms:

> *Lumbar pain caused by the fei yang vessel shows a swelling on the painful spot or irritability with pain. If it gets worse, people become afraid and sad. For this lumbar pain, insert a needle five divisions above the internal ankle, this is the point feiyang, in front of the kidney meridian, at the meeting place of the yin wei mai.*[90]

This is usually seen as KI-9.[91]

The *Nan Jing's* descriptions are more clearly of an emotional nature:

> *For yang wei mai disease there is {both a physical and emotional} suffering of cold or heat symptoms. . . {For} yin wei mai disease, there is {both a physical and emotional} suffering of heart pain symptoms.*[92]

The *Nan Jing* further explains the emotional relationship:

> *Yin and yang cannot balance; the {visible} emotions will be thinking too much, obsession, loss of will and lack of self control.*[93]

Wang Shu He makes some important theoretical statements about the wei mai:

> *Yang is wei {protecting}, this controls the surface. Wei is qi. The yang accepts the evil, the disease stays at the surface, but not at the lining. Cold and heat bother the patient.*
> *Yin is ying {nourishing}, ying is blood, the heart is {controls} the blood, which is why the patient is bothered by heart pain.*[94]

This reconfirms the relationship of the triple warmer and pericardium and the surface, wei qi, and lining, ying qi, through their luo points, TW-5 and PC-6, the treatment points of the yang and yin wei mai.

In a yang wei mai problem, the pulse will be floating with symptoms of brief eye dizziness, yang excess, difficulty breathing, needing to raise the shoulders to breathe, feelings of coldness.[95] In a yin wei mai problem, the pulse will be big and full with symptoms of pain in the chest, feelings of fullness at the sides of the body below the ribs accompanying heart pain. In males, if the yin wei pulse feels like a "ball passing beneath the fingers," there will be accompanying symptoms of feelings of fullness at the sides of the ribs and pain in the lumbar area. In females, this will have the accompanying symptom of a pain in the sexual organ that feels like a wound or injury.[96]

Zhen Jiu Ju Ying — Yin and Yang Wei Mai Treatments

Treat PC-6 then SP-4 for:

- full condition with discomfort on the inside: heart, stomach
- shanghan: master of the heart
- stagnation and fullness in the heart and chest: liver, stomach
- irregular vomiting: spleen, stomach
- feeling of fullness in the chest {pressure in the heart caused by a deficient, damp spleen with mucus}: lung, heart
- abdominal pain: stomach
- watery diarrhea or frequent loose stools: large intestine
- alcohol mucus, stagnant pain in the upper part of the middle warmer {painful, rebellious, full condition with bad smelling belches}: master of the heart
- inability to transform rice and grains: stomach
- lump in the inguinal crease {or severe muscle tension between the scapulae, or severe tension at the side of the navel, caused by cold wind invading the uterus}: liver, stomach
- anal prolapse in children: master of the heart
- pain in the sides and rib cage: liver, gallbladder
- blood stabbing pain in women: heart, liver
- borborygmus: large intestine

- lump pain: liver
- in males, problem below the ribcage on one side caused by alcohol: spleen, lung
- "two diaphragm" {a feeling of fullness and distension around the diaphragm} and stagnation below the sternum {with lump and pain}: heart, spleen, stomach
- diaphragm qi and food cannot pass {stagnation in the throat and esophagus causing difficulty swallowing, the feeling of something rising and bad smelling belches}: stomach, heart, lungs
- heart and ribcage swollen and painful: spleen, stomach, master of the heart
- intestine wind and bleeding from the anus: large intestine
- shanghan knot in the chest {evil qi is knotted in the chest, when the knot appears it causes pain below the sternum that is tight on palpation}: stomach
- anus painful following a bout of diarrhea: small intestine
- stagnant food at the diaphragm: master of the heart, stomach[97]

Treat TW-5 then GB-41 for:

- swelling and pain of the four limbs and joints: kidney
- arms cold and painful: triple warmer
- epistaxis: lung
- heat of the hands and feet: triple warmer
- inability to stretch or bend the fingers with joint pain: triple warmer
- pain in the bone around the eyes {caused by external wind heat, mucus, dampness stagnating between the eyebrows, possibly rhinitis or sinusitis}: bladder
- pain in the hands and feet: stomach
- dread of wind after labor: kidney, stomach
- shanghan, injury by cold with spontaneous sweating: stomach, lungs
- head wind: bladder
- inability to move the four limbs smoothly: gallbladder, stomach
- muscle, tendon or bone pain: liver, kidney

- tearing in a wind: liver
- sore, red eyes: liver, heart
- swelling and pain of the lumbar and back: kidney
- numbness, pain and weakness of the arms and legs: stomach
- swollen eyes: heart
- head wind with shaking and pain: bladder
- shanghan, injury by cold with superficial fever: bladder
- tetanus: liver, stomach
- pain of the hand and arm: large intestine, triple warmer
- pain of the head and back of the neck: small intestine
- night sweating: master of the heart
- shadow on the eyes {cataract}: liver
- body swollen after labor: stomach, kidney
- pain in the lumbar area and hip joint: kidney
- thunder head wind: gallbladder[98]

Zhen Jiu Da Cheng Yin and Yang Wei Mai Treatments

The *Zhen Jiu Da Cheng* gives the following treatments for the two pairs of points.

For the yin wei mai, PC-6 can balance diseases of the heart, gallbladder, spleen and stomach. PC-6 and SP-4 together can treat:

- a feeling of fullness, stagnation and swelling inside the chest and the heart
- borborygmus
- watery diarrhea
- anal prolapse
- difficulty swallowing because of diaphragm stagnation, with further damage when alcohol is consumed
- a hard, tight (yin) lump at the sides of the body in the abdomen in women, the lump is painful, with heart pain
- knot in the chest (pain below the sternum, heart) that feels tight and full on palpation
- after much diarrhea, the anus is painful and spasming

- the feeling of a knot, tightness or pain in the chest associated with shanghan
- nue disease

For the yang wei mai, TW-5 controls wind, cold, muscular luo {superficial diseases that affect the muscles} and skin diseases. TW-5 and GB-41 together can treat:

- joints of the four limbs swollen and painful with coldness of the knees
- cold knees
- inability to raise the four limbs with head wind
- bone or muscle problems of the back and groin
- pain on the head, back of the neck and around the eyes
- hands and feet hot and numb with night sweats
- red, swollen and infected eyes {associated with tetanus}
- shanghan with spontaneous sweating, the patient feels hot superficially[99]

Zhen Jiu Da Cheng
Yin and Yang Wei Mai Combination Treatments

The *Zhen Jiu Da Cheng* gives the following combination treatment schedules for the yin wei mai and yang wei mai.

Yin wei mai treatment combinations:

- feeling of fullness and discomfort {in the middle warmer} associated with shanghan and discomfort in the stomach {stomach flu}: PC-6 and CV-12, PC-7, ST-36, CV-17
- middle warmer feels full and stagnant with stabbing pains at both sides of the ribs: PC-6 and TW-6, LV-13, CV-17
- spleen and stomach have deficient cold symptoms, vomiting and nausea: PC-6 and ST-44, CV-12, CV-6, SP-4

- spleen and stomach qi deficient {weak digestion}, heart and abdomen swollen and full: PC-6 and SP-3, ST-36, CV-6 and CV-9
- pain at the lower lateral edges of the ribs, stabbing pain inside the stomach and heart: PC-6 and CV-6, LV-2, GB-34
- stagnation or lump that will not disperse, deep pressure pain in the heart: PC-6 and PC-7, CV-12, SP-6
- stagnant food that will not disperse, slow wasting of the body: PC-6 and SI-3, BL-20, SP-4
- increasing congestion of food (imbalance between the spleen and stomach with fullness around CV-12 that is uncomfortable to the touch, constipation and acid regurgitation), lump caused by bleeding, hidden {deep} pain in the abdomen: PC-6 and BL-20, LV-2, CV-6
- five kinds of yin organ lumps or qi lumps {fluid or gas lumps in the intestines}, or blood lumps {with fixed sharp pain} on one side of the abdomen causing stagnation of food: PC-6 and BL-17, BL-18, LV-1, KI-6
- yin and yang organs deficient and cold, both sides of the body painful: PC-6 and TW-6, HT-5, BL-20, GB-34
- congealed, stagnant qi, easily loses control, too much thinking, melancholic, sad, stabbing pain in the heart and abdomen: PC-6 and BL-12, CV-17, PC-8, ST-36
- large intestine deficient and cold, anal prolapse: PC-6 and GV-20, GV-4, GV-1, BL-57
- difficulty passing stools, straining to pass stools causing anal prolapse: PC-6 and KI-6, GV-20, TW-6
- organ poisoning, swollen pain, blood in the stools that does not stop: PC-6 and BL-57, BL-18, BL-17, GV-1
- five kinds of hemorrhoids, the pain feels as if it is on the outside: PC-6 and BL-55, GV-1, BL-57
- five kinds of epilepsy, bubbly saliva in the mouth: PC-6 and SI-3, HT-7, BL-15, gui yan, SP-1 LU-11 bilaterally and simultaneously.
- "heart type" of idiot, unending sadness and crying: PC-6 and HT-5, SI-3, HT-7, KI-4
- madness, "heart surprised," cannot distinguish friend or foe: PC-6 and HT-1, HT-9, BL-15, CV-12, shi xuan

- forgetfulness, mental unclarity (like senility): PC-6 and BL-15, HT-5, HT-9
- heart qi deficient or lost, laughing or singing, the patient seems to be losing their mind: PC-6 and HT-4, BL-15, HT-5
- "heart surprised," babbling, speech unclear: PC-6 and HT-3, HT-8, BL-15, SI-3
- deficiency in the heart, paranoid all the time, shen and thinking are anxious: PC-6 and ST-18, HT-5, BL-15, BL-19
- "heart surprised," leading to collapse and coma: PC-6 and PC-9, GV-20, LV-1
- heart and gallbladder deficient, attacked by shock, surprise, upset, or stress causing palpitations: PC-6 and HT-6, BL-15, HT-5
- heart deficient and gallbladder cold, whole body shivering: PC-6 and BL-19, HT-5, GB-41[100]

The poetic descriptions of some of the emotional symptoms require some explanation. "Easily loses control" indicates that the patient easily becomes angry or emotional. The "heart type" of idiot is someone who is idiotic and displays heart syndrome symptoms. "Heart surprised" is used to indicate that the heart suffers from nervous shock perhaps severe enough to lead to collapse and coma; this may be a shock-induced cerebrovascular accident or cardiac infarction.

To treat SP-1 and LU-11 bilaterally and simultaneously the procedure recommended was to tie the toes together and moxa SP-1 at both sides. Then, tie the thumbs together and moxa LU-11 in tandem.

Yang wei mai treatment combinations:

- both arms, from the shoulders down, are red and swollen, joints sore: TW-5 and LI-12, LI-15, SI-4
- redness, swelling and pain of the internal ankle bone: TW-5 and KI-3, GB-40, GB-41, BL-60
- finger joints painful, unable to bend or stretch: TW-5 and SI-4, SI-5, LI-4, wu hu
- toe joint pain, unable to walk: TW-5 and ST-44, LV-3, BL-60

- congested, knotted heat of the five yin organs, vomiting blood: TW-5 and BL-13, BL-15, BL-17, BL-18, BL-20, BL-23
- congested, knotted heat of the six yang organs, reckless blood: TW-5 and BL-17, BL-19, BL-21, BL-22, BL-25, BL-27, BL-28
- epistaxis that does not stop, reckless bleeding: TW-5 and SI-1, BL-15, BL-17, KI-1
- vomiting blood, dizziness, unconsciousness, almost comatose: TW-5 and BL-18, BL-17, HT-5, LV-1
- weakness, no energy, rebellious qi, vomiting blood that does not stop: TW-5 and BL-38, BL-17, dantian {the area around CV-4, CV-5, CV-6}, BL-18
- vomiting blood, epistaxis, yang overcomes the yin, hot blood, reckless blood: TW-5 and PC-9, BL-18, BL-17, ST-36, SP-6,
- cold blood, vomiting blood, yin overcomes the yang (vomiting blood is related to the heart and lung meridians): TW-5 and LU-11, BL-15, HT-7, BL-13, BL-17, SP-6
- tightness, stiffness of the tongue, difficulty speaking, white buds on the tongue: TW-5 and TW-1, PC-9, CV-24, juquan
- heavy, swollen puffy tongue, very high fever, unable to speak: TW-5 and shi xuan, haiquan, jin jin, yu ye
- sore or abscess inside the mouth: TW-5 and GV-27, TW-6, CV-24, shi xuan
- vomiting that will not stop ("strong yang"): TW-5 and KI-1, GV-27, HT-9, HT-7
- tongue contracted, difficulty speaking ("strong yin"): TW-5 and BL-15, CV-17, haiquan
- lips split and bleeding, dryness and soreness of the skin of the lips: TW-5 and CV-24, LU-11, TW-1
- lump on the neck {such as tuberculosis in the lymph nodes of the throat. Usually lung and kidney yin deficient related, it begins at bean size and is without pain, then enlarges and becomes painful, sometimes filling with pus}: TW-5 and TW-10, GB-20, zhou jian, ST-12, shi xuan
- lump that extends from the front of the chest down to the armpit {tuberculosis of the lymph nodes}: TW-5 and GB-21, CV-17, PC-7, TW-6, GB-34

- swelling near the left ear lobe, on palpation one can feel a knot or lump inside {tuberculosis of the lymph nodes}: TW-5 and TW-17, SI-3, zhou jian
- swelling near the right ear lobe, on palpation one can feel a knot or lump inside {tuberculosis of the lymph nodes}: TW-5 and TW-17, ST-6, SI-3, LI-4
- earlobe red, swollen and painful: TW-5 and LI-4, TW-17, ST-6
- redness and swelling of the neck that will not go away: TW-5 and GV-16, GB-21, CV-24
- infection of the surface of the eyes {conjunctivitis}, unable to open the eyes: TW-5 and BL-1, LI-4, BL-18, shi xuan
- following exposure to wind, the eyes are swollen, itchy and tearing: TW-5 and BL-2, TW-23, LI-2, xiao gukong
- following exposure to wind, the eyes are red, swollen, spots in the eyes, small pimples of flesh appear on the outer canthi of the eyes: TW-5 and TW-22, BL-1, BL-2, BL-18, BL-54, LI-4, zhou jian, KI-6, LU-7, shi xuan
- toothache, both sides of the chin swollen and painful: TW-5 and GV-26, LI-4, lu xi
- pain in the upper canine teeth, unable to open the mouth: TW-5 and LU-9, ST-6, LI-4, lu xi
- pain in the lower canine teeth, cheeks and neck red and swollen: TW-5 and LI-5, CV-24, ST-6, KI-3
- deafness, qi stagnation and pain in the ear: TW-5 and GB-2, BL-23, ST-36, TW-17
- ringing, itchiness or soreness in the ear: TW-5 and GB-3, LI-4, GB-2
- thunder head wind, dizziness, fullness in the chest, pressure in the heart with diaphragm problems {caused by spleen deficient mucus or damp spleen}: TW-5 and GV-20, CV-12, LU-9, BL-12
- deficient kidney headache, heavy head, unable to lift the head: TW-5 and BL-23, GV-20, KI-3, LU-7
- "mucus rebellious head and eye dizziness," vertigo: TW-5 and LV-1, BL-18, GV-20
- pain on the top of the head: TW-5 and GV-23, GV-20, GB-19, KI-1, LI-4
- eyes red, painful, hot: TW-5 and BL-2, LI-4, LI-20[101]

"Yang overcomes the yin" would refer to an excess of yang overwhelming yin. "Mucus rebellious head and eye dizziness" would mean a severe dizziness caused by mucus obstruction.

Dr. Yang's Yin and Yang Wei Mai Treatments

- spasms and numbness following apoplexy: TW-5 and TW-3, TW-4, LI-11, ba xie.[102]

Treatment Point Locations

Point locations for the eight extraordinary vessel treatment points are consistent. In classical and modern Japanese and Chinese texts, SP-4, PC-6, TW-5, SI-3, GB-41, KI-6 and BL-62 have all been similarly located. LU-7 is the only point to have variant locations. It appears that these discrepant locations are the result of different interpretations of an abstruse location technique.

LU-7 is either placed one and a half divisions proximal to the wrist crease behind the styloid process of the radius, between the radius and the radial artery, or one and a half divisions proximal to the wrist crease behind the styloid process of the radius, but in a small hollow on the radius. The second method places it closer to the large intestine meridian. The earliest descriptions, those of the *Zhen Jiu Jia Yi Jing,* place this point just one and a half divisions proximal to the wrist crease without any further specification. However, by the time of the *Tongren Shu Xue Zhen Jiu Tu Jing* of the eleventh century, a new method of location had been developed. This involved finding the point at the end of the forefinger, while holding the thumb of the opposite hand in the palm, with the second, third and fourth fingers (at the back of the hand). The forefinger can either be held on a line that places it in the small hollow on the radius, or on a line that places it on the LU-9, LU-8, LU-6 aspect of the lung meridian.

In the classical texts the location intended is not clear. In modern China, consensus places LU-7 in the small hollow on the radius. In Japan, consensus places the point between radius and radial artery. Thus, when using modern Japanese treatment techniques, we suggest using the location between the radius and radial artery. To resolve the problem of locating LU-7 for the classical treatments, we suggest using palpation. In our experience, when

LU-7 needs treatment, the location between the radius and radial artery will be sore. If not, check the second location.

SP-4 is located on the medial aspect of the foot one division behind the big toe joint, slightly inferior to the first metacarpal bone.

PC-6 is located two divisions proximal to the wrist crease between the two central tendons on the palmar side of the forearm.

SI-3 is found with the hand held loosely in a fist, just behind the head of the fifth metacarpal bone.

TW-5 is located on the dorsal surface of the forearm, two divisions proximal to the wrist crease between the radius and ulna.

GB-41 is located at the point of junction of the fifth and fourth metatarsal bones on the dorsum of the foot.

BL-62 is located slightly below the inferior margin of the external malleolus (some say in a depression).

KI-6 is located one division directly below the medial malleolus.

Extra Point Locations

The point locations that follow may be found in various books. We have used: *Acupuncture, A Comprehensive Text, Book of Acupuncture Points,* and the *Zhen Jiu Jing Wai Qi Xue Tu Du,* a modern Chinese extra point book.

Bai lao is located two divisions above and one division lateral to GV-14, on both sides.

Ba xie refers to four points on each hand. These are found with the hand in a clenched fist, between the heads of each of the metacarpal bones.

Du yin is located on the underside of each of the second toes in the middle of the second crease.

The eyes of the knee, xi yan, are found with the knee flexed. They are in the hollows either side of the patellar tendon below the kneecap.

The location of the extra point "above the throat" is unclear, though its meaning is likely a sore point found above the larynx.

Gui yan refers to the bilateral, simultaneous treatment of SP-1 and LU-11 with the thumbs and big toes bound together.

Hai quan is located on the underside of the tongue in the center of the frenum linguae.

Jin jin is found on the underside of the tongue with the tongue rolled back, at the vein to the left of the vinculum linguae.

Points Under
The Tongue

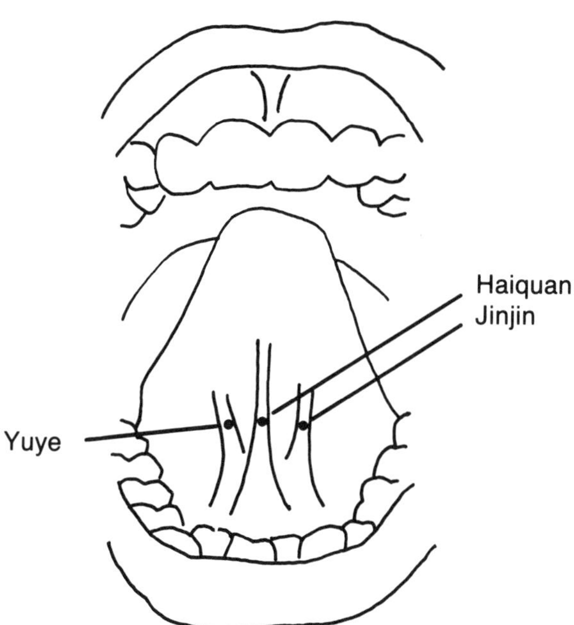

Figure 20

Ju quan is found on the upper surface of the tongue, in the center of the dorsum.

Lu xi is located on the superior surface of the internal malleolus.

Shi xuan refers to ten points, on the middle of the tip of each finger about 0.1 divisions from the finger nail.

Tai yang lies on the temple about one division behind the mid point between the outer canthus of the eye and tip of the eyebrow.

Tian ying is a reactive point similar to an ah shi point. It refers to the reactive point that feels comfortable with and is relieved by pressure.

Wu hu refers to points on the knuckles of the index and ring fingers.

Xiao gu kong lies at the dorsal aspect in the middle of the transverse crease of the phalangeal joint of the little finger.

Yin tang is the mid point between the two eyebrows.

Yu ye is found on the underside of the tongue with the tongue rolled back, at the vein to the right of the vinculum linguae.

Zhong kui lies on the dorsal aspect at the tip of the bone on the proximal phalangeal joint of the middle finger.

Zhou jian lies at the prominence of the olecranon when the elbow is flexed.

Point Indication Summaries

Point indications in the classical sources used are also consistent. The *Zhen Jiu Ju Ying* and the *Zhen Jiu Da Cheng* give nearly identical information in almost all cases. These two books drew their information extensively from the *Zhen Jiu Jia Yi Jing* (282 AD), the *Tongren Shu Xue Zhen Jiu Tu Jing, Bronze Statue Textbook* (1027 AD) and the *Ming Tang* text contemporary to the *Su Wen*. The *Ming Tang* is referred to only in the older books and is no longer extant.

LU-7 Indications	
Zhen Jiu Da Cheng	**Zhen Jiu Ju Ying**
Needle: 0.2 div. remove after 5 exhalations disperse for 5 inhalations *Moxa*: 7X	*Needle*: 0.2 div. remove after 3 exhalations disperse for 5 inhalations *Moxa* 7-49X
Main Effects	
hemiplegia, face	hemiplegia, face and arm
hand and arm without energy	
hemiplegia of the body	
heat in the palms	heat in the palms
inability to open mouth	inability to open mouth
nue	nue
vomiting bubbly saliva	vomiting bubbly saliva
cough	cough
incessant laughing	incessant laughing
split lip	split lip
forgetfulness	forgetfulness
blood in the urine	blood in the urine
pain in penis	pain in penis
urine feels hot	urine feels hot
epilepsy	epilepsy
abscess of the face, eyes or four limbs	abscess of the face, eyes or four limbs
shoulder bi	shoulder bi
chill of chest and back	chest and back cold, shivering
shortness of breath	shortness of breath
rebellious symptoms, falls down corpse-like, caused by cold or heat	corpse-like cold symptoms
confused, distressed, clen- ching hands or unclear vision	

In a full condition: chest and back hot, sweating, four limbs swollen
In a empty condition: chest and back chilled (and shaking – *Ju Ying*), shortness of breath.[103]

SP-4 Indications	
Zhen Jiu Da Cheng	**Zhen Jiu Ju Ying**
Needle: 0.4 div. *Moxa*: 3X	*Needle*: 0.4 div. *Moxa*: 3X
Main Effects	
cold nue	cold nue
no appetite	no appetite
pre-epileptic condition	pre-epileptic condition
sighing	sighing
too much nue and sweating	too much nue and sweating
if the disease peaks, nausea occurs; if vomiting occurs, the disease subsides	if the disease peaks, nausea occurs; if vomiting occurs, the disease subsides
head and face swollen	head and face swollen
heart anxious and mentally disturbed	heart anxious and mentally disturbed
excess alcohol, gallbladder empty	excess alcohol, gallbladder empty
rebellious qi rising, causing overexcitement	rebellious qi rising, causing over excitement

If full condition: there will be stabbing pain in the intestines, disperse the point.

If empty condition: the abdomen will be swollen, tonify the point.[104]

SI-3 Indications	
Zhen Jiu Da Cheng	**Zhen Jiu Ju Ying**
Bronze: *Needle*: 0.1 div. *Moxa*: 1X	*Bronze*: *Needle* 0.1 div. *Moxa*: 1X tonify if small intestine deficient
Main Effects	
nue	nue
red eyes with vision problems	red eyes with cataract problems
epistaxis	epistaxis
full condition of the chest	full condition of the chest
skin problem that results in hard scabby skin	skin problem that results in hard scabby skin
back and neck stiff, tight	head and neck stiff, tight
inability to turn head	inability to turn head
epilepsy	epilepsy
spasming and tightness of elbow and arm	spasming and tightness of elbow and arm
deafness	deafness[105]

BL-62 Indications	
Zhen Jiu Da Cheng	**Zhen Jiu Ju Ying**
Bronze: *Needle*: 0.3 div. *Moxa*: 3X	*Bronze*: *Needle*: 0.3 div. *Moxa*: 3X
Main Effects	
wind dizziness	wind dizziness
lumbar and leg pain	lumbar pain
thighs weak, cannot stand for long	thighs weak, cannot stand for long
completely exhausted	completely exhausted
rebellious qi, cold qi	rebellious qi, cold qi
lumbar and iliac cold bi	lumbar and iliac cold bi
difficulty bending, stretching legs, knees	difficulty bending, stretching legs, knees
blood, qi pain, gynecological problems	blood, qi pain, gynecological problems
daytime epilepsy (moxa)	daytime epilepsy (moxa)[106]

KI-6 Indications	
Zhen Jiu Da Cheng	**Zhen Jiu Ju Ying**
Su Wen commentary: *Needle*: 0.4 div. *Moxa*: 3X	*Su Wen* commentary: *Needle*: 0.4 div. *Moxa*: 3X
Bronze: *Needle*: 0.3 div. *Moxa*: 7X	*Bronze*: *Needle*: 0.3 div. *Moxa*: 7X
Main Effects	
dry throat	dry throat
heart sad, unable to enjoy things	heart sad, unable to enjoy things
four limbs weak and tired	four limbs weak and tired
chronic nue	chronic nue
acute pain in testicles with swelling (caused by cold contraction in the liver meridian) or of the lower abdomen or back	acute pain in testicles with swelling (caused by cold contraction in the liver meridian) or of the lower abdomen or back
nausea, vomiting	nausea, vomiting
wants to lie down	wants to lie down
"big wind," pain moving	"big wind," pain moving
seeing stars (spots in eyes)	
lower abdominal pain	lower abdominal pain
rebellious menstruation	rebellious menstruation
cannot control four limbs	
penis always erect or itching	penis always erect or itching
turbid discharge from penis (and vagina?)	turbid discharge from penis (and vagina?)
pain on one side of the lower abdomen with discharge	pain on one side of the lower abdomen with discharge
irregular menses	irregular menses
vaginal prolapse	stretched penis (possibly hernia)
nighttime epilepsy (moxa)	nighttime epilepsy (moxa)[107]

PC-6 Indications	
Zhen Jiu Da Cheng	**Zhen Jiu Ju Ying**
Bronze: *Needle*: 0.5 div. *Moxa*: 3X	*Bronze*: *Needle*: 0.5 div. *Moxa*: 3X
Main Effects	
wind heat in hand	wind heat in hand
loss of will	loss of will
heart pain	heart pain
red eyes	red eyes
elbow spasm	elbow spasm

If full condition: there will be violent pain in the heart, disperse the point.

If empty condition: the head will be stiff and tight, tonify the point.[108]

TW-5 Indications	
Zhen Jiu Da Cheng	**Zhen Jiu Ju Ying**
Bronze: *Needle*: 0.3 div. *Moxa*: 2X	*Bronze*: *Needle*: 0.3 div. *Moxa*: 2X
Ming Tang: *Moxa*: 3X	*Ming Tang*: *Moxa*: 3X
Main Effects	
deafness	deafness
pain in five fingers, unable to grasp things	pain in five fingers, unable to grasp things

If full condition: the elbow will spasm; disperse the point.

If empty condition: the elbow will be loose; tonify the point.

To treat this point, the arm should be neither stretched nor bent[109]

GB-41 Indications	
Zhen Jiu Da Cheng	**Zhen Jiu Ju Ying**
Jia Yi Jing: *Needle*: 0.2 div. *Moxa*: 3X	*Jia Yi Jing*: *Needle*: 0.2 div. *Moxa*: 3X
Main Effects	
full feeling in chest	full feeling in chest
large abscess from ST-12 to armpit	large abscess from ST-12 to armpit
bites cheeks easily	bites cheeks easily
swelling around TW-16	swelling around TW-16
wanton sexual desire	
thighs weak with no energy	
eye dizziness	eye dizziness
occipital bone pain	occipital bone pain
cold and chill	cold and chill
heart pain	heart pain
wandering bi symptoms	wandering bi pain
rebellious qi and panting	rebellious qi and panting
irregular menses	irregular menses
ribcage full and painful	ribcage full and painful
abscess on breast	abscess on breast
	daily nue[110]

Correspondences to Modern Terminology

We have stated that the *Zhen Jiu Da Cheng* treatment combinations appear to be similar to later syndrome differentiations and treatments that are in common use today. The following are a few examples:

Syndrome Correspondences		
Syndrome	**Symptoms**	**Treatment Points**
Lung Qi Deficient, Wind Invasion	attacked by wind; susceptible to cold; coughing; panting	LU-7, CV-17, BL-12, LI-4, GV-16
Spleen Qi Deficient	swollen abdomen and umbilicus with undigested food (in the stools)	SP-4, ST-25, CV-9, ST-44
Spleen Qi Deficient	whole body weak; no energy in the four limbs	GB-41, bai lao, BL-15, ST-36, CV-4, BL-38
Deficient Yin	heat in the "five hearts"	KI-6, PC-6, KI-1, shi xuan, PC-7, LI-4, BL-17, BL-19
Excess "Zhong Feng" obstructed organ succumbing to wind	four limbs spasming after stroke	BL-62, LI-12, LI-9, LU-10, GB-31, LV-7, SP-6
Excess "Zhong Feng" obstructed organ succumbing to wind	tension of body, eyes rolled into head after stroke	BL-62, GV-20, bai lao, LI-4, LV-2, LI-11, shi xuan, GB-34
Hot Blood	epistaxis that won't stop, reckless bleeding	TW-5, SI-1, BL-15, BL-17, KI-1
Hot Blood	vomiting blood; epistaxis; yang overcomes yin; hot blood; reckless bleeding	TW-5, PC-9, BL-18, BL-17, ST-36, SP-6

Notes

[1] Techniques and methods of palpation are discussed extensively in *Hara: Reflections on the Sea.*

[2] *Zhen Jiu Da Cheng,* p. 191.

[3] *Ibid.*

[4] This reference can be found in the *Zhen Jing Zhi Nan, Zhen Jiu Ju Ying* and *Zhen Jiu Da Cheng.*

[5] These were referred to in the *Su Wen.* The *Zhen Jing Zhi Nan* uses the older character found in the *Su Wen,* the *Zhen Jiu Ju Ying* uses a slightly simplified character, both of which refer to the same practice. These references tend to support the argument that extraordinary vessel theory and treatment evolved from Daoist tradition.

[6] *Zhen Jing Zhi Nan,* p. 165; *Zhen Jiu Ju Ying,* p. 149.

[7] *Ibid.,* p. 156; *Zhen Jiu Ju Ying,* p. 143.

[8] *Zhen Jiu Ju Ying,* p. 149.

[9] *Nan Jing,* Chapter 28, vol. 2, p. 15, based on *Su Wen,* Chapter 60.

[10] Wang Shu He, *Commentary on the Nan Jing,* vol. 2, p. 15.

[11] Wang Shu He, *Commentary on the Nan Jing,* vol. 2, p. 14.

[12] In *Hara: Reflections on the Sea* we discuss the differentiation of palpable abdominal masses according to *Nan Jing* five element theory.

[13] *Mai Jing,* vol. 2, p. 16.

[14] *Zhen Jing Zhi Nan,* pp. 162-163 *passim; Zhen Jiu Ju Ying,* pp. 147-148 *passim.*

[15] *Zhen Jiu Da Cheng,* p. 187.

[16] See *Su Wen,* Chapter 35.

[17] Waichi Sugiyama, *Sugiyama Ryu Sanbusho,* p. 10. Shohaku Honma, *Shinkyu Byosho Gaku,* p. 129.

[18] Shohaku Honma, *Shinkyu Byosho Gaku,* pp. 129-130.

[19] Sorei Yanagiya, *Kanmei Humon Shinsatsu Ho,* p. 359.

[20] Shohaku Honma, *Shinkyu Byosho Gaku,* pp. 129-130.

[21] Waichi Sugiyama, *Sugiyama Ryu Sanbusho,* p. 10.

[22] Shohaku Honma, *Shinkyu Byosho Gaku,* pp. 129-130.

[23] Sorei Yanagiya, *Kanmei Humon Shinsatsu Ho,* p. 359.

[24] Shohaku Honma, *Shinkyu Byosho Gaku,* pp. 129-130.

[25] Sorei Yanagiya, *Kanmei Humon Shinsatsu Ho,* p. 359.

[26] *Su Wen,* Chapter 35.

[27] See for instance: Sugiyama and Honma.

[28] Shohaku Honma, *Shinkyu Byosho Gaku,* pp. 129-130.

[29] Waichi Sugiyama, *Sugiyama Ryu Sanbusho,* p. 10.

[30] *Ibid.*

[31] See *Hara: Reflections on the Sea* for additional discussion of the relationship of the triple warmer to water function.

[32] *Zhen Jiu Da Cheng,* pp. 187-189.

[33] *Ibid.*

[34] *Ling Shu,* Chapter 33, p. 281 *passim.*

[35] *Ibid.,* p. 282 *passim.*

[36] See Mr. Ito's treatments in the next chapter.

[37] *Ling Shu,* Chapter 65, pp. 463-4.

[38] *Nan Jing,* Chapter 29, vol. 2, p. 17.

[39] Wang Shu He, *Commentary on the Nan Jing,* vol. 2, p. 17.

[40] Li Shi Zhen, *Qi Jing Ba Mai Kao,* vol. 1, p. 15. Gao Wu, *Zhen Jiu Ju Ying,* pp. 133-134.

[41] Wang Shu He, *Mai Jing,* vol. 2, p. 16 *passim.*

[42] *Ibid.*

[43] Li Shi Zhen, *Qi Jing Ba Mai Kao,* vol. 1, p. 15.

[44] Gao Wu, *Zhen Jiu Ju Ying,* pp. 133-134 *passim.*

[45] *Zhen Jing Zhi Nan,* pp. 156-157 *passim; Zhen Jiu Ju Ying,* p. 143 *passim.*

[46] *Zhen Jiu Da Cheng,* p. 179.

[47] *Ibid.*, pp. 179-181.

[48] *Ibid.*

[49] *Jinkui Yaolue Fanglun,* quoted from Li Shi Zhen, *Qi Jing Ba Mai Kao,* vol. 1, p. 23.

[50] *Su Wen,* Chapter 60, p. 321.

[51] Li Shi Zhen, *Qi Jing Ba Mai Kao,* vol. 1, p. 22.

[52] *Nan Jing,* Chapter 28, vol. 2, p. 14.

[53] Wang Shu He, from the *Mai Jing,* quoted from Li Shi Zhen, *Qi Jing Ba Mai Kao,* vol. 1, p. 23.

[54] The commentator of the *Nei Jing Jie Po Sheng Li Xue,* p. 119.

[55] Wang Shu He, *Mai Jing,* vol. 2, p. 16 *passim.*

[56] *Zhen Jing Zhi Nan,* pp. 160-161 *passim; Zhen Jiu Ju Ying,* p. 146 *passim.*

[57] *Zhen Jiu Da Cheng,* p. 182.

[58] *Ibid.*, pp. 182-183.

[59] *Ibid.*

[60] Wang Shu He, *Commentary on the Nan Jing,* vol. 2, p. 15.

[61] *Nan Jing,* Chapter 28, vol. 2, p. 15.

[62] Wang Shu He, *Mai Jing,* vol. 2, p. 16 *passim.*

[63] Li Shi Zhen, *Qi Jing Ba Mai Kao, vol. 1, p. 24.*

[64] *Zhen Jing Zhi Nan,* pp. 158-159 *passim; Zhen Jiu Ju Ying,* pp. 144-145 *passim.*

[65] *Zhen Jiu Da Cheng,* p. 184.

[66] *Ibid.*, p. 185.

[67] *Ibid.*

[68] *Su Wen,* Chapter 63, p. 346.

[69] *Ling Shu,* Chapter 21, p. 215.

[70] *Nei Jing Jie Po Sheng Li Xue,* p. 132.

[71] *Su Wen,* Chapter 41, p. 233.

[72] *Ling Shu,* Chapter 23, p. 233.

[73] Li Shi Zhen, *Qi Jing Ba Mai Kao,* vol. 1, p. 7.

[74] *Nan Jing,* Chapter 29, vol. 2, p. 17.

[75] Wang Shu He, *Commentary on the Nan Jing,* vol. 2, p. 17 *passim.*

[76] *Ibid.*

[77] Wang Shu He, *Mai Jing,* vol. 2, p. 16 *passim.*

[78] *Nei Jing Jie Po Sheng Li Xue,* p. 132.

[79] Li Shi Zhen, *Qi Jing Ba Mai Kao,* vol. 1, p. 9.

[80] *Zhen Jing Zhi Nan,* pp. 161-162 *passim; Zhen Jiu Ju Ying,* p. 147.

[81] *Ibid.*, pp. 163-164 *passim; Zhen Jiu Ju Ying,* pp. 148-149 *passim.*

[82] The *Zhen Jiu Da Cheng,* p. 189 (yin qiao mai); p. 183 (yang qiao mai).

[83] *Ling Shu,* Chapter 63 p. 439, discusses how sweetness affects the spleen, promoting worms.

[84] *Zhen Jiu Da Cheng,* pp. 189-190.

[85] *Ibid.*

[86] *Ibid.*, pp. 183-185.

[87] *Ibid.*

[88] *Su Wen,* Chapter 41, p. 230.

[89] *Huang Di Nei Jing Tai Su,* vol. 10, p. 155.

[90] *Su Wen,* Chapter 41, p. 230.

[91] *Zhen Jiu Jia Yi Jing,* from *Nei Jing Jie Po Sheng Li Xue,*, p. 143.

[92] *Nan Jing,* Chapter 28, vol. 2, p. 15.

[93] *Ibid.*, Chapter 29, vol. 2, p. 17.

[94] Wang Shu He, *Commentary on the Nan Jing,* vol. 2, p. 15.

[95] Wang Shu He, *Mai Jing,* vol. 2, p. 15.

[96] *Ibid.*

[97] *Zhen Jing Zhi Nan,* pp. 157-158 *passim; Zhen Jiu Ju Ying,* pp. 143-144 *passim*

[98] *Ibid.*, pp. 159-160 *passim; Zhen Jiu Ju Ying,* pp. 145-146 *passim.*

[99] *Zhen Jiu Da Cheng,* p. 181 (yin wei mai); p. 185 (yang wei mai).

[100] *Ibid.*, pp. 181-182.

[101] *Ibid.*, pp. 185-187.

[102] *Ibid.*

[103] *Zhen Jiu Ju Ying,* p. 13, *Zhen Jiu Da Cheng,* p. 6.

[104] *Ibid.*, p. 40, *Zhen Jiu Da Cheng,* p. 23.

[105] *Ibid.*, p. 51, *Zhen Jiu Da Cheng.* p. 31.

[106] *Ibid.*, p. 72, *Zhen Jiu Da Cheng,* p. 43.

[107] *Ibid.*, p. 80, *Zhen Jiu Da Cheng,* p. 48.

[108] *Ibid.*, p. 87, *Zhen Jiu Da Cheng,* p. 53.

[109] *Ibid.*, p. 92, *Zhen Jiu Da Cheng,* p. 56.

[110] *Ibid.*, p. 107, *Zhen Jiu Da Cheng,* p. 65.

[111] Editor's note: There is considerable similarity between the *Da Cheng* locations and symptomologies and Tin Yau So's descriptions. See: Tin Yau So, *Book of Acupuncture Points.*

Extraordinary Vessels

Modern Extraordinary Vessel Treatments

An excellent way to learn the use of the extraordinary vessels is to examine the work of practitioners who use these vessels exclusively, or extensively. Ms. Michi Tokito uses the extraordinary vessels exclusively with excellent results.[1] Her treatments involve a differentiation of the relative excess or deficiency of the yin and yang of the body at the level of the triple warmer, the master of the heart, ming men. Based on this assessment, she places zinc and copper plated needles in combinations designed to balance these essential energies.

The treatments formulated by Ms. Tokito are root treatments, working at the deepest level of the body where yin and yang begin to manifest. They demonstrate how the extraordinary vessels may be used to reach the root levels of the energetic system and how the more complex theoretical relationships may be applied in practice. Her exclusive use of the extraordinary vessels, coupled with the use of gradient generating metals, is a clear indication that these vessels are indeed related to bioelectrical biases and subtle currents. In clinical application, it is important to bear in mind that these treatments are total treatments. When using these procedures, no other treatments or therapies should be done.

The second practitioner we feature is Mr. Osamu Ito, who uses the extraordinary vessels extensively, though not exclusively. By applying a sophisticated adjunctive therapy that uses a complex diagnostic style, his treatments demonstrate how the extraordinary vessels my be integrated with local treatments and other systems of acupuncture.[2] His treatments manifest the topological, structural nature of the extraordinary vessels. Field effects and the sensitivity of these vessels to magnetic influences are also evident when examining his results. Mr. Ito's treatments utilize the polarity of the north and south magnetic poles and the gradient potentials of gold and aluminum. Combining these two stimuli, north with gold and south with aluminum, placement of the magnets or metals on the appropriate extraordinary vessel treatment points can correct structural stresses and deformities that obstruct energetic function.

Another technique employed by Mr. Ito consists of north and south pole magnets connected to an electric stimulator that directs measured pulses to the magnets. These treatments are also root treatments, though they are often used with local treatments. His results support the idea that local treatments are more effective when performed after, or in conjunction with, root treatments. In a clinical setting, these procedures offer the added benefit of non-invasive treatment as an adjunct to the routine acupuncture treatment.

In both of these featured treatment styles, the practitioner's attention is directed to signs rather than symptoms. The patient's presenting complaints are considered as guides or confirmation of the assessment of total condition. Symptoms are considered in the secondary assessments that modify the primary treatment or determine the adjunctive therapy. The body itself is the source of the most important information. In learning these styles you will find you are considering many subtle observations that are easy to overlook: leg length differences, color changes, muscle tension and point sensitivity. Almost all the asymptomatic styles require this detailed investigation of the body, demanding considerable skill in your palpatory and observational diagnosis. It is here that the thorough study of extraordinary vessel theory and pathways reaps full benefit. Looking for a sign a little to the left or right, a little higher or lower, or at an alternate location, may be all that is required to complete the diagnostic picture.

These two treatment styles can teach us much about the use of the extraordinary vessels. They do not, of course, exhaust the use of the extraordinary vessels in acupuncture practice. Dr. Manaka's ion cords, the Chinese and European methods of insertion acupuncture are also effective. All these systems demonstrate two important points about the use of the extraordinary vessels. The theory of these vessels, the various pathways and the classical treatments strongly imply that the extraordinary vessels function through gradients. The techniques that have evolved in practice are heavily weighted toward polarity stimulation. The ion cords, the electrical potentials of different metals, the polarity of magnets and the right to left polarities that are featured in extraordinary vessel treatment styles also hint that biases are a major element of extraordinary vessel function.

In the ion cord treatments unidirectional ion flow is the stimulus created. With Ms. Tokito's system the various metals used to coat the needles have electrical potentials, the "circuit" that allows these potentials to become electrical energy is the extraordinary vessel treated. The same principles are involved in Mr. Ito's use of magnets and electrically pulsed magnets. In China today, while it is often taught that the master and coupled points are needled bilaterally, this is not the only type of treatment applied. There are many styles in Europe; some teach needling bilaterally, others contralaterally and others ipsilaterally. In England the use of different potentials is not often discussed, yet polarities based on gender and other factors are often used. The gender based polarities are similar to the left—right, male—female distinctions made by the *Zhen Jiu Da Cheng.*[3]

The second pattern that is clear in these treatment systems is the pervasive combination of extraordinary vessel points with local treatment points. The structure of these treatments is an extraordinary vessel treatment supplemented by points that have a direct effect on the presenting problem. While this is not surprising in the modern treatments, since the technique is well accepted in China and Japan through the work of Nagatomo, Manaka, Ito and others, it is interesting to find the same structure in the *Zhen Jiu Ju Ying* and the *Zhen Jiu Da Cheng*. In the *Zhen Jiu Da Cheng*, for example, we find the following treatment recommended:

Tension, hardness, tightness in head and back of neck	
Point	**Use**
SI-3	Root treatment
CV-24, GV-16, GB-20	Local points
LI-4	Effect on the problem area

The pattern is found again in treatment of the following conditions:

Deep stabbing pain in chest	
Point	**Use**
SP-4, PC-6	Root treatment
PC-7	Effect on the heart
KI-26	Local point

Poisoning on dorsum of hand	
Point	**Use**
BL-62	Root treatment
TW-2, TW-3, LI-4, TW-5	Local points

The pattern is found again in the *Zhen Jiu Ju Ying* treatment examples:

Toothache	
Point	**Use**
GB-41 then TW-5	Root treatment
Do Yin exercise	Root treatment
If needed, LI-11 or ST-36	Local treatment

Here, LI-11 and ST-36 are chosen because of the pathways of the stomach and large intestine meridians.

Stagnant Throat	
Point	**Use**
SI-3 then BL-62	Root treatment
Do Yin exercise	Root treatment
If needed, ST-36, KI-10 or LU-5	Local treatment

Again, the adjunctive points are selected because of the pathways of the stomach, kidney and lung meridians.

Eyes Tear in the Wind	
Point	**Use**
TW-5 then GB-41	Root treatment
Do Yin exercise	Root treatment
If needed, LV-8	Local treatment

Because the liver controls the eyes, LV-8 is the adjunctive point.

As a working premise, we may consider the extraordinary vessels as a deep internal network of bioelectrical pathways. Stimulation of that network potentializes or enhances the energetics of the body. Thus, the local treatments applied may function freely, without the impediment of functional or structural obstruction. Awareness of these patterns helps to organize our study.

Tools and Principles

The use of two or more needles made of different metals is a modern phenomenon. The different metals produce electrical currents in the body in addition to the effects that result from the insertion of needles. The use of north and south magnetic poles produce similar electrical phenomena. Colloquially, these materials create an electro-acupuncture effect of natural currents. In Asia, Mr. Tsugio Nagatomo, one of Mr. Ito's teachers, pioneered this field. His work was in part stimulated by the research of Dr. Yoshio Manaka, and by the work of several European practitioners, among them Gerhard Bachmann, whose developments seem to have been particularly influential to Mr. Nagatomo's work.[4] Based on the research of these practitioners, a "minus—plus needles" school of acupuncture has developed. Many treatments utilizing zinc and copper plated needles, needles of other metals and the placement of metals directly on the skin have been developed. In the West there is considerable interest in these therapies, in part because of the Western history of "magnetic therapies" and in part because of the apparent newness of the idea; however, most of the English language information is considerably understated. The qualities of the metals or magnets are used entirely within the diagnostic and therapeutic principles of Oriental medicine.

When two different metals are placed on the body, small electrical currents are induced, similar to the operative principle of a battery. This property is based on the relative electrical properties of each of the metals. Physically, this depends on the ease of ionization of the outer shell of electrons in the atoms of the metals. Stainless steel, zinc and aluminum are dispersing or cold. Silver and copper are mildly tonifying. Gold is the most tonifying and warming. The following chart briefly summarizes the electrical properties of the metals. The upper part of the chart includes the more negative metals: aluminum (Al), zinc (Zn), nickel (Ni). Tin (Sn) is the only neutral metal. At the bottom of the chart are copper (Cu), silver (Ag), gold (Au). These are positive and tonifying.[5]

Metal	Symbol	Quality
Lithium	Li	Most negative
Potassium	K	
Calcium	Ca	
Sodium	Na	
Magnesium	Mg	
Aluminum	Al	
Zinc	Zn	
Chromium	Cr	
Ferrous (divalent) iron	FeII	
Cadmium	Cd	
Cobalt	Co	
Nickel	Ni	
Tin	Sn	Neutral
Lead	Pb	
Ferric (trivalent) iron	FeIII	
Copper	Cu	
Mercury	Hg	
Silver	Ag	
Gold	Au	Most positive

The different metals used in practice are usually selected for both electrical potential and the practicality of use. Mr. Nagatomo uses zinc, copper, tin and cobalt needles; Ms. Tokito, copper and zinc; Mr. Ito, gold and aluminum. The principle is simultaneous use of a metal from the negative side of the scale and one from the positive side of the scale: copper—zinc, gold—aluminum. This polarity induces electrical and ionic currents. The further apart on the scale, the larger the currents. Thus, copper and zinc will create a smaller current than gold and aluminum. Both combinations are effective with different treatment styles. Mr. Ito combines the use of north—south magnetic polarity with the gold and aluminum metal pair.

Metal polarity treatments are not exclusive to the extraordinary vessels. However, the principles of operation change when treating the twelve meridians. When treating the extraordinary vessels, the master point receives copper, gold or the north magnet; the coupled point receives the zinc, aluminum or south magnetic pole. On the twelve meridians, when treating a painful or sensitive area (an excess indication), zinc, aluminum or the north magnetic pole are used. A distal point, or a deficient meridian, takes the copper, gold or south facing magnet. Thus, *the polarity reverses when not using the extraordinary vessels.* This is often confusing. It demonstrates that the extraordinary vessels have different polar qualities than the twelve meridians, a relationship that has been experientially and clinically verified.[6]

Point Selection

When using Ms. Tokito's treatments, the following combinations of points and metals are used:

Combination One		
Point	**Master/Coupled**	**Metal**
Left PC-6	master yin wei mai	copper
Right BL-62	coupled yang qiao mai	zinc
Left SP-4	coupled chong mai	zinc
Right SI-3	master du mai	copper

Combination Two		
Point	**Master/Coupled**	**Metal**
Left TW-5	master yang wei mai	copper
Right KI-6	coupled yin qiao mai	zinc
Left GB-41	coupled dai mai	zinc
Right LU-7	master ren mai	copper

Combination Three		
Point	**Master/Coupled**	**Metal**
Right TW-5	master yang wei mai	copper
Left KI-6	coupled yin qiao mai	zinc
Right GB-41	coupled dai mai	zinc
Left LU-7	master ren mai	copper

In Mr. Ito's treatments the following point, metal and magnet combinations are used:

Combination One			
Point	**Master/Coupled**	**Metal**	**Magnetic Pole**
SI-3 (bilateral)	master du	gold	north
BL-62 (bilateral)	coupled yang qiao	aluminum	south

First Adjunct to Combination One			
Point	**Master/Coupled**	**Metal**	**Magnetic Pole**
Left or right SP-4	master chong	gold	north
Left or right PC-6	coupled yin wei	aluminum	south
Left or right N-I	finger, yin wei	aluminum	south

Second Adjunct to Combination One			
Point	**Master/Coupled**	**Metal**	**Magnetic Pole**
KI-6 (bilateral)	master yin qiao	gold	north
LU-7 (bilateral)	coupled ren	aluminum	south
N-II (bilateral)	finger, yin qiao	aluminum	south

Third Adjunct to Combination One			
Point	**Master/Coupled**	**Metal**	**Magnetic Pole**
Left or right TW-5	master yang wei	gold	north
Right or left GB-41	coupled dai	aluminum	south
Left or right P-I	finger, yang wei	gold	north

The points N-I, N-II, and P-I are special points, their location is discussed later in the text.

In addition to the induced electrical stimulation provided by magnets and electrically complementary metals, another reason that Mr. Ito has applied magnets in his treatments relates to the body's sensitivity to both weak and strong magnetic fields. In particular, the body is sensitive to the geomagnetic field, as it helps establish and maintain many biological functions and rhythms. While researching the cause of clinically nondefinable diseases, Dr. Kyoichi Nakagawa found that people are often not sufficiently exposed to the geomagnetic field.[7] Problems associated with such underexposure are: backache, stiff shoulders, discomfort around the neck and shoulders, headache, heaviness of the head, insomnia, constipation, heaviness of the legs, dizziness, unidentified chest pain, tiredness of the whole body, psychological problems.

Dr. Nakagawa named this the "magnetic field deficiency syndrome." It is closely associated with features of modern lifestyle. People who drive frequently, live or work in highrise buildings or buildings with steel superstructures, are particularly prone to this condition. His research found that magnets can be applied to the body to relieve many of these problems. This research and the mounting evidence of the biological effects of magnetic fields provide another part of the theoretical background of magnet therapies and help to explain how the application of magnets can have such powerful effects.

Needle Technique

For Ms. Tokito's treatments, the zinc and copper plated needles that are used are very small and require the use of a special insertion tube or tweezers. These needles are always angled horizontally; insertion places them just through the skin, 1-2 millimeters deep, 2-3 millimeters maximum. No additional stimulation technique is required. The direction of insertion is important: the needles are angled toward heaven (when standing with hands above the head). Thus, on the legs, the needles are directed toward the body; needles on the arms are directed toward the hands. If tweezers are used to insert the needles, the following procedure is used:

Step	**Action**
1:	Locate the exact point to be treated.
2:	Hold the needle near to the needle head, and position the tip just over the point, almost flush with the skin.
3:	Pull the skin slightly away from the point of the needle.
4.	Press the needle, gently, tip down into the skin.
5:	Hold the needle steady, slowly release the skin allowing it to rise over the needle.
6:	Use the tweezers to adjust the depth of insertion.

When using the small insertion tube, the following procedure is followed:

Step	**Action**
1:	Slide the needle handle first into the tube.
2:	Place the end of the tube on the point, keeping the tube flush with the skin.
3:	Angle the tube slightly into the point.
4:	Depress the head of the insertion tube; the shaft of the tube should barely touch the head of the needle.
5:	Use two or three gentle taps on the handle to insert the needle. Be careful not to insert too deeply.
6:	Insert or withdraw the needle to the correct depth.

Zinc and copper needles are difficult to sterilize completely. We recommend beginning with new needles and keeping each set of two zinc and two copper needles in each patient's file, maintaining the records necessary to insure that the needles are used for one patient only.

Magnets

Mr. Ito uses small six hundred gauss magnets that he designed, the "Ito" magnet. The north pole is painted green, with a piece of gold at the core, and is denoted "N^{600}." The south pole is painted white, with a piece of aluminum at the core, and is denoted "S^{600}." The adjunctive therapy magnets are three thousand gauss magnets embedded in a synthetic, electrically conductive element to which electrodes may be attached. Mr. Ito uses a pointer electric machine, a device equipped with four south and four north magnets, the south magnets having a "dimple" in the face. The waveform and strength of the current directed to the magnets is designed for his treatment style. References to applying current to magnets therefore presume the use of this machine. When using the magnets, place them face (metal side) down on the point and secure with first aid paper tape. The same procedure is used for the three thousand gauss magnets. Attach the clips of the cords from the pointer machine, red to north denoted "$(N)^{-3000}$" and black to south denoted "$(S)^{-3000}$." Place tape over both the magnet and clip. Zinc and copper balls in conjunction with 600 gauss or stronger magnets may be used in place of the Ito magnets. Zinc is combined with the south pole and copper with the north pole. It is best to tape the zinc and copper on the points, then tape the magnet on top of the tape at the side of the metal ball. This insures that the zinc and copper make contact with the skin without interference from the metal of the magnet.

Use of the pointer machine is simple. After the magnets have been attached with the cord, slowly increase the setting of the outlet used until the patient recognizes the pulsing sensation. Generally, patients feel a light pulsing or tingling. The stimulation should be light and comfortable. On most parts of the body this will require an intensity setting of four. For exceptionally sensitive people or small children a lower setting is likely. Insensitive areas will require a higher intensity, sometimes as high as nine or ten on the intensity dials. All magnets should be placed before stimulating any of the magnets. All should receive the same length of stimulation, up to twenty minutes. If the strength of the electrical stimulation increases subjectively, adjust the intensity until the patient feels that it is close to the original level. If the patient becomes insensitive, increase the stimulation to the original level.

When using the pointer machine, there are certain conditions and contraindications that should be followed. The machine should always be preset to a "constant" stimulus, at a frequency setting of two and at the low frequency level. These settings are suitable for electromagnet therapy. When switching the connections on, begin at the "two' setting; the red light should start flashing. Then, slowly increase the setting until the patient begins to feel the stimulation. Always recheck pressure pain, the sensitivity of the point or area where the north facing magnet has been placed after three or four minutes of stimulation. If the reaction has decreased substantially, continue treatment. If it has changed somewhat, wait and recheck the indications shortly. If there is little or no change, or in rare cases, if the significant points or areas have become more sensitive, it is necessary to relocate the south facing magnet according to the applications described in the text. Without rechecking and relocating where appropriate, the treatment will be ineffective.

Contraindications for the use of the electro-magnetic pointer machine therapy:

- ✔ Patients with lowered white blood cell counts;
- ✔ Pregnant women;
- ✔ Patients using a pacemaker;
- ✔ Patients with very high blood pressure;
- ✔ Very elderly patients;
- ✔ Very fatigued patients;
- ✔ Patients who are suffering from a heart problem at the time of the treatment, for example, angina;
- ✔ Patients with a "cold" or "flu," an external invasion disease, at the time of the treatment;
- ✔ Patients with metal allergies;
- ✔ Patients with a skin condition or other problem in the area where the magnets should be placed;
- ✔ Patients for whom electrical stimulation is onerous.

If the patient has allergies to metals, the reactions usually only appear from extended application or retention of magnets. The twenty minutes of pointer machine use is insufficient to trigger the reactions. However, there are some patients with severe allergies for whom this manner of treatment is not advised.

Because many of these treatments utilize only the small electrical currents created by the polarities of the magnets and different metals, it is important that all other metal in contact with the body be removed. This includes rings, earrings, bracelets, chains, belts and watches. Tights, hosiery and other synthetic clothing should be removed since these fabrics have electrostatic effects. Throughout treatment, the patient should remain quiet, warm and still.

Tokito
Triple Warmer — Ming Men
Balancing Treatments

These are simple treatments, based exclusively on the finding that the deep chi (foot) pulse of the right side (pericardium, master of the heart, ming men) is weaker or stronger than the deep chi pulse of the left side (kidney). The positional pulse diagnosis of the *Nan Jing* is used.[8] Ms. Tokito theorizes that all disease results from an imbalance between the triple warmer and pericardium, master of the heart, ming men. All disease comes from an imbalance at the level of the essential, basic energetic dualities. This is a difficult concept to understand, for Ms. Tokito is gauging energies at the level that they become the specific meridian qi.

Ming men, master of the heart lies at the back of the body. According to tradition it is at the side of the second lumbar vertebra or below the second lumbar vertebra, the location of the acupoint ming men. The body's energies focus here and are projected forward to the triple warmer, which has its source in the moving qi between the kidneys.[9] Thus, the energies are projected to the triple warmer in the area between the kidneys. Here the transformations that produce each of the specific energies take place. Prenatal qi from the kidneys and heart, qi from breath, food and fluids and the biorhythmic energies of the cosmos focus, blend and transform in the abdomen.

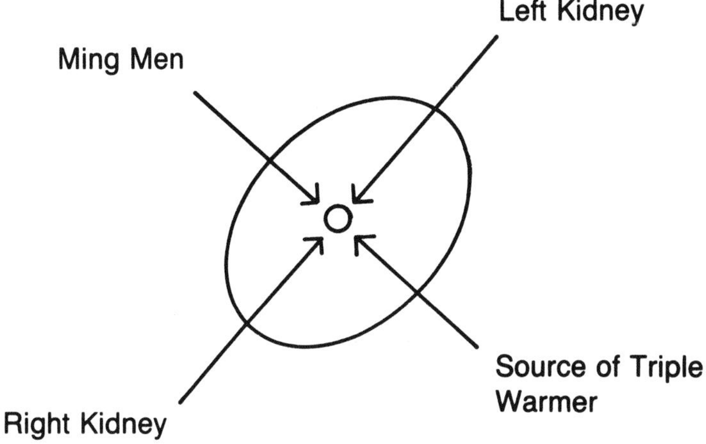

Moving Qi Between the Kidneys

Figure 21

This stepping down and focussing of energies is the transformation from no-form to form. The moving qi maintains the vital transformations and is the "pivot" of the triple warmer and the kidneys;[10] hence triple warmer deficiencies are measured in the kidney pulse. Imbalances of the triple warmer and master of the heart, ming men reflect in imbalances in the moving qi between the kidneys. Since three of the extraordinary vessels have their origins and roots in the moving qi, the extraordinary vessels provide a means for accessing deep imbalances. This is what Ms. Tokito's treatments accomplish. Her diagnosis is completely asymptomatic, the treatment is conceived without regard for the presenting symptoms. Thus, the pulse diagnosis used is extremely important.

One should carefully compare the relative strength of the left deep pulse in the chi position with the right deep chi position pulse:

Step	Action
1.	Use your usual pulse procedure. If there appears to be a difference in the right and left deep guan pulses, continue; if not, the treatment is not appropriate.
2.	Arrange the patient so that you may check the pulses at both wrists simultaneously.
3.	Use the index, middle and ring fingers, slowly and gently press to the bone.
4.	Note how easily and quickly the pulses disappear.
5.	Raise the fingers from the bone, slowly and gently.
6.	Note how quickly and easily the pulses reappear.
7.	Check each side alternately, use steps 3, 4, 5 and 6.
8.	Check each side together, use steps 3, 4, 5 and 6.

It is best to take both pulses at the same time with the patient lying down, arms folded over the abdomen. Generally, taking the pulse in a sitting position is acceptable for gauging pulse quality but it is not accurate enough for gauging these subtle strength differences. When there are obvious differences in strength, Ms. Tokito's treatments may be used. However, when the difference is not so obvious, incorrect diagnosis is easy; do not use this treatment. It is also necessary to palpate the sternocleidomastoid muscles to assess their relative tension. When treatment is correctly applied these muscles will relax. Knowing their condition prior to treatment allows you to monitor how treatment has progressed.

The treatment procedure utilizes two copper and two zinc needles and is applied in four steps. The first step includes the insertion of a copper needle to one point and a zinc needle to another, according to the sequence indicated by the pulse. The second step requires that the pulse is repeatedly rechecked. If diagnosis and point location are accurate, the relative strength of the pulse in the right and left deep chi position will equalize and the sternocleidomastoid muscles will relax. This will take a few minutes, sometimes only one or two; the pulse should be checked and rechecked during this time. The third step commences when the pulses equalize. Insert the other copper and zinc needles according to the specified sequence. In the fourth, and final, step, all four needles are left in place for ten to twenty minutes then removed in reverse order. Needles are retained no less than ten minutes and no more than twenty minutes. They can be removed when the reactive areas on the body are less reactive or when the patient becomes less relaxed.

If you have palpated other areas of the body, the knees, abdomen, mu or back shu points, as part of your diagnosis, you should repeat these palpations after treatment. Often, many of these points will be less reactive, and can exhibit remarkable changes. The greater the change, the more appropriate the treatment and the quicker the relief.

In each treatment only four points are used, two on the left and two on the right. Once you have determined the treatment to use, it is important that the points are located as accurately as possible. Needle technique must be correct, do not hurry through the procedure. Always palpate the four points chosen to ascertain the exact point to be treated. Sometimes the reactive area is very small. In these cases, use a small probe such as a "teishin" to find the exact sore point for needle insertion.

Tokito Weak Ming Men Pulse Treatment

If the kidney pulse, left chi pulse, is stronger than the right chi pulse, this indicates a weak ming men condition. The following points are treated in the sequence given:

Series	Side	Point	Needle	Vessel
First series	Left	PC-6	Copper	yin wei mai
First series	Right	BL-62	Zinc	yang qiao mai
Second series	Left	SP-4	Zinc	chong mai
Second series	Right	SI-3	Copper	du mai

Remember to insert the two needles of the first series first. Then, check the pulses and sternocleidomastoid muscles. When the chi pulses equalize, treat the two points of the second series.

Tokito Weak Kidney Pulse Treatment

If the ming men pulse, right chi pulse, is stronger than the left chi pulse, this indicates a weak triple warmer condition. The point selection for this treatment is determined by a distinction between the left and right superficial bar pulses, the gallbladder and stomach pulses. These are the pulses felt with slight pressure in the bar position. If you cannot differentiate the strength of the stomach and gallbladder pulses, the treatment is not appropriate.

If the gallbladder pulse is stronger than the stomach pulse use the following points in the sequence given:

Series	Side	Point	Needle	Vessel
First series	Right	TW-5	Copper	yang wei mai
First series	Left	KI-6	Zinc	yin qiao mai
Second series	Right	GB-41	Zinc	dai mai
Second series	Left	LU-7	Copper	ren mai

If the stomach pulse is stronger than the gallbladder pulse, use the following points in the sequence given:

Series	Side	Point	Needle	Vessel
First series	Left	TW-5	Copper	yang wei mai
First series	Right	KI-6	Zinc	yin qiao mai
Second series	Left	GB-41	Zinc	dai mai
Second series	Right	LU-7	Copper	ren mai

Practitioners who are able to make fine pulse differentiations are able to use this treatment protocol almost all the time with great success; beginners should use the technique only when the pulse data is clear. Since the treatment addresses a fundamental element of energetic balance, it is able to have profound effects in a variety of conditions. Like "open points" and other deep, root treatments, the presenting problem is secondary; it is usually at a more superficial level. Our experience with patients indicates that abdominal reactions that would have taken several treatments to ameliorate may clear in a single treatment.

Ms. Tokito's treatments diagnose and treat imbalances of yin and yang at the primary level of their manifestation in the body, as can be seen in the following diagrams. The eight extraordinary vessel points were described in connection with the eight trigrams in the temporal sequence, the later heaven sequence:

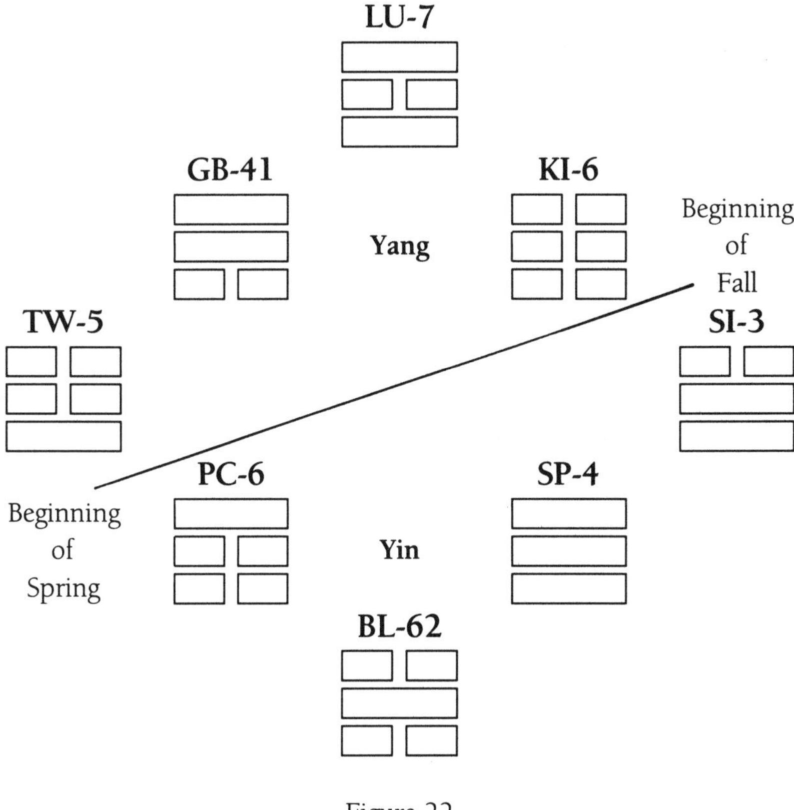

Figure 22

The treatment for triple warmer deficiency treats the four points above the line; the treatment for ming men deficiency treats the four points below the line. On the left, the line coincides with the beginning of spring, on the right, with the beginning of fall. The trigrams above this line represent the yang aspect of the yearly cycle; those below the line are the yin aspect.

In effect, Ms. Tokito is using the extraordinary vessels to access and equalize the yin and yang of the body at the deepest level, at the point where the human energy system meets, joins and is differentiated from the generalized energies of the universe. Theoretically, this is the energetic strata that underlies all the energetic dualities of the body. In a deficient triple warmer and thus water—kidney condition, the triple warmer is tonified. In a deficient fire—master of the heart, ming men condition the pericardium, master of the heart is tonified.

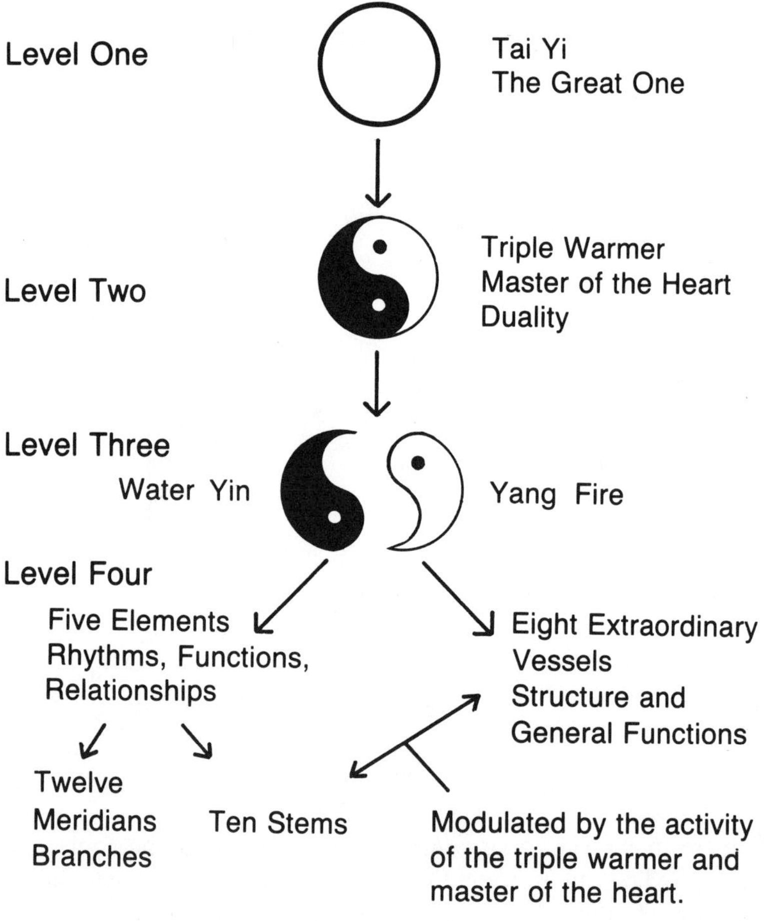

Figure 23

The treatment of triple warmer and kidney deficiency involves tonifying the triple warmer through treating TW-5 and KI-6 with an electric gradient. The weak ming men treatment tonifies the master of the heart through treating PC-6 and BL-62 with an electric gradient. The treatments access energies at level two before the energies are differentiated to level three, thus balancing the energies at levels three and four. This perspective is based on a model we have extrapolated from the classical literature; the triple warmer and master of the heart have "a name but no form" and represent the first manifestation of the energies that stem from the abdomen, the moving qi between the kidneys. Since this energetic root lies roughly at the center of gravity, it is affected by and affects the structure of the body. Once again, this underscores the topological—energetic nature of the extraordinary vessels, helping us understand how they produce structural and energetic changes.

We should remember that Ms. Tokito, a practical person, arrived at her treatment procedures through many years of clinical practice and observation. Their real strength lies in practice. Her greatest theoretical interest is the synthesis of the extraordinary vessel and element—stem models. By diagnosing and treating these simultaneously, the deepest root imbalance, that of triple warmer and master of the heart, ming men, may be corrected.

Ito Structural Balance Treatments

Mr. Ito considers the energetics of the body relative to the correct structure of the body. Having studied both bone manipulation and acupuncture, he realized that the knees, lower back (particularly the sacrum) and the neck were vitally important in correcting structure and energetic function, and thus in controlling and treating disease. These three areas are essential to the balance and health of the spine, which is important to the correct function of many systems in the body. With this as a fundamental premise, he used palpation and treatment to determine clinical rules. He discovered that the use of zinc, copper and magnets, and later, gold, aluminum and magnets on the extraordinary vessels, corrected structural imbalances. Through experience he devised a simple means for diagnosing and confirming the use of pairs of extraordinary vessels. Particularly, he discovered correspondence points on the knees, lower back and sacrum.

Mr. Ito has also recorded correlations of symptoms to each of the extraordinary vessel pairs. These differ from classical symptomologies and the indications for using ion cords on the extraordinary vessels.[11] In his style of treatment, diagnosis is based on compilations of data from examination of the body's structure and on palpation of the knees and lower back. The indications found determine the pairs of extraordinary vessels that will be connected with metal and magnet stimulation on the corresponding master and coupled points. Diagnosis of the knees involves sliding the thumbs rapidly back and forth with light pressure, then with firmer pressure, on the following areas:

Vessels	**Procedure**
Yin Qiao Mai and Ren Mai	The medial edge of the knee, level with the lower border of the patella.
Yin Wei Mai and Chong Mai	The area around the medial aspect of the eyes of the knee.
Yang Wei Mai and Dai Mai	The area around the lateral aspect of the eyes of the knee.

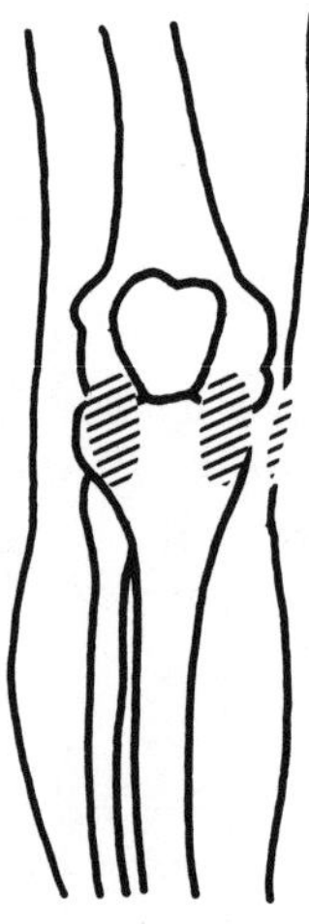

Figure 24

In each of these areas pressure pain, puffiness, swelling, tightness, knots, palpable ligaments or tendons or any unusual sensation is an indication for treatment of the corresponding vessel pair. To confirm the diagnosis or to differentiate the most relevant area, if more than one area is reactive, the lower back is also palpated. Palpation should be performed with the patient lying on their abdomen. Pressure pain or tension found between lumbar vertebrae L2 and L3, L3 and L4 or L4 and L5 indicate the chong mai to yin wei mai connection. The most significant area is lumbar vertebrae L3 to L5. Pressure pain or tension on BL-23, BL-33, or BL-32 and josen (between lumbar L5 and sacral S1) indicate the ren mai to yin qiao mai connection. Pressure pain or tension at the lateral and superior corners of the sacrum indicates the dai mai to yang wei mai connection. These areas are also therapeutically useful· with Mr. Ito's adjunctive therapy.

Vessels	Procedure
Yin Qiao Mai and Ren Mai	Palpate for pressure pain, tension or any unusual sign on BL-23, BL-33, BL-32 and josen.
Yin Wei Mai and Chong Mai	Palpate for pressure pain, tension or any unusual sign between L2, L3, L4, L5. The most significant are L3 to L5.
Yang Wei Mai and Dai Mai	Palpate for pressure pain, tension or any unusual sign at the lateral and superior corners of the sacrum.

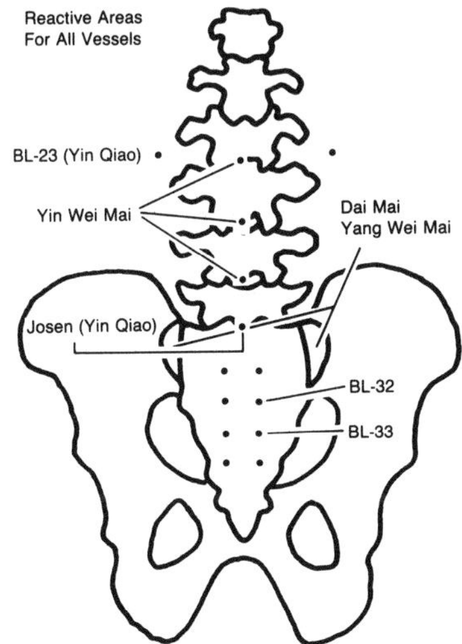

Figure 25

Mr. Ito reports the following symptom complexes. The yin wei mai to chong mai connection is confirmed by:

- presence of palpable tension, soreness, tightness, discomfort below the ribs at the subcostal region (chest distress)
- stomach or duodenal ulcer
- strained back
- knee pain
- heart problems
- palpitations
- shortness of breath
- intercostal neuralgia
- herpes zoster
- sciatica that shoots down to the big toe passing through the inside of the leg, around the spleen meridian.

For the yin qiao mai to ren mai connection one may find symptoms of:

- sciatica that runs down the bladder meridian
- headache
- insomnia
- cold feet
- stiff shoulder
- high blood pressure
- gynecologic problems
- nephritis
- nephrosis
- cystitis
- asthma
- whiplash injury
- cold lumbar area
- Meniere's syndrome.

For the yang wei to dai mai connection one may find symptoms of:

- one leg longer than the other (have the patient lie on their abdomen, pull the legs gently towards you, while the patient keeps their head on the midline and then compare the heels)

- eagle toes (the toes are curved over and clawed)
- sciatica that runs down the gallbladder meridian
- backache
- migraine
- tinnitus
- trigeminal neuralgia
- stiff shoulder
- any problem or discomfort that is one sided.

The key signs and symptoms for the chong mai, yin wei mai are illustrated as follows. Palpation reaction will accompanied by symptoms of ulcers, intercostal neuralgia, heart problems and knee pain:[12]

Reactive Back Area — Chong & Yin Wei Mai

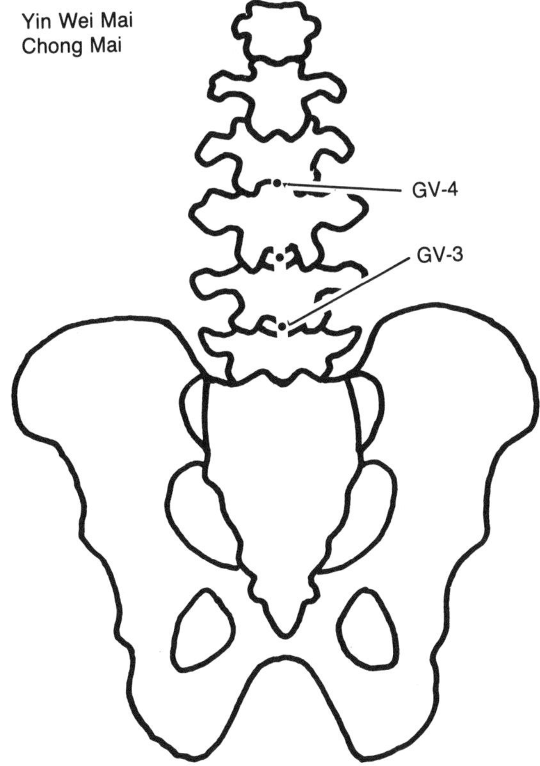

Figure 26

Reactive Knee Area — Chong & Yin Wei Mai

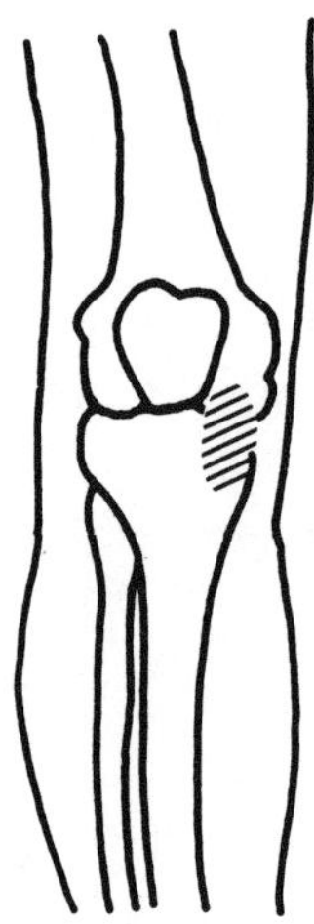

Figure 27

The key signs and symptoms for the dai mai, yang wei mai are illustrated in the following manner:

Reactive Back Area — Dai & Yang Wei Mai

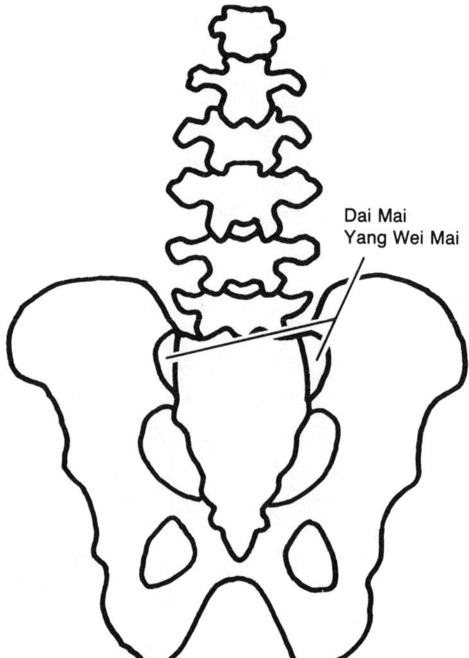

Figure 28

Reactive Knee Area — Dai & Yang Wei Mai

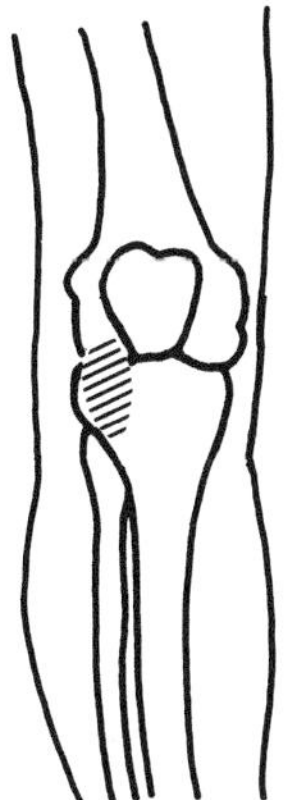

Figure 29

Palpation reaction will be accompanied by one sided complaints and difference in leg length. This sign reflects imbalances in the three most important areas, the knees, neck and sacrum. Usually, treatment will correct the leg length difference, a necessary procedure to undertake whenever such discrepancy is noted.

The key signs and symptoms for the yin qiao mai, ren mai are illustrated in the following manner:

Reactive Back Area — Ren & Yin Qiao Mai

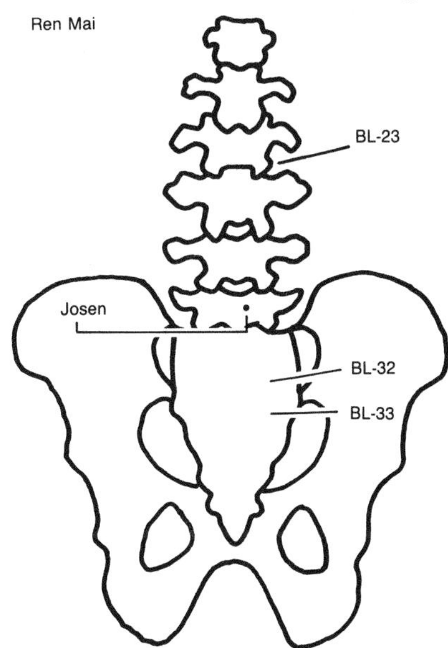

Figure 30

Reactive Knee Area — Ren & Yin Qiao Mai

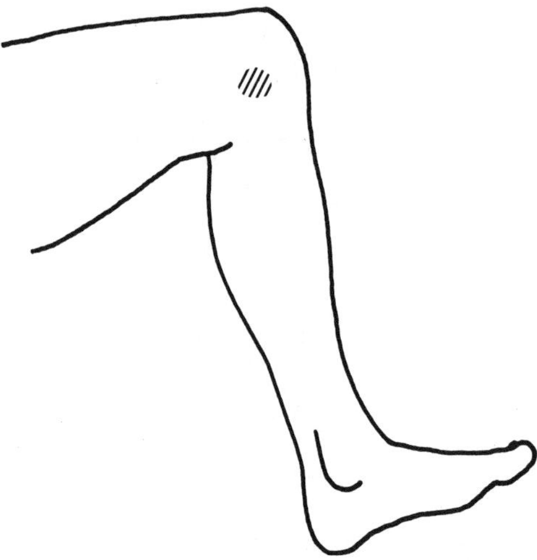

Figure 31

Palpation reaction will be accompanied by gynecological problems or feelings of coldness in the lower body.

Special Point Locations

In more recent research, Mr. Ito has developed and refined his treatment procedures to use the special extraordinary vessel reflex points located on the middle fingers. These were discovered by Mr. Ito from his further study of a unique system of hand acupuncture developed by a Korean practitioner, Dr. Tae Woo Yoo.[13] These points reflect the yang wei, P-I, yang qiao, P-II, yin wei, N-I and yin qiao, N-II. P-I is located on the laterodorsal side of the middle fingers, midway between the corner of the nail and the end of the crease of the first joint. P-II is located at the same level on the medial side.

Right Middle Finger

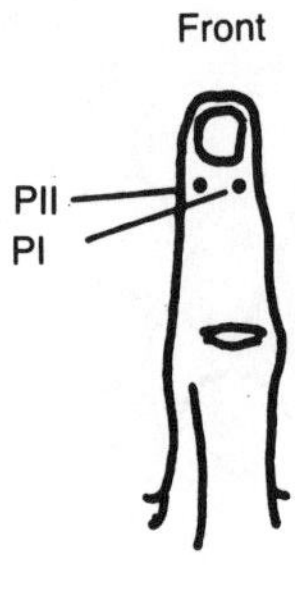

Figure 32

N-I is located at the same level as P-I, directly opposite P-I on the lateropalmar side of the middle fingers; N-II is located at the same level, directly opposite P-II.

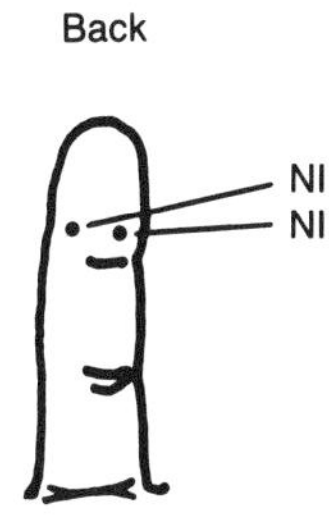

Figure 33

P-II is generally not used in these treatments, and is included only for reference. P-I is always treated with north facing magnets, the N^{600}, while N-I and N-II are always treated with south facing magnets, S^{600}. Either a north or south magnet is added to the appropriate points, while magnets are placed on the extraordinary vessel meridian points.

Treatment Procedures

Similar to Ms. Tokito's treatments, there is a twenty minute maximum for the application of the Ito magnets. Adhere to this limit strictly. For all three treatments, points corresponding to the extraordinary vessel diagnosed are used in combination with BL-62 and SI-3 bilaterally. Mr. Ito has found that optimum results are obtained when treating yin wei mai, yang wei mai or yin qiao mai in combination with the du mai and yang qiao mai, due to the added effect of treating the spine with BL-62 and SI-3. In all treatments, aluminum and south pole magnets are bilaterally applied to BL-62, gold and north pole magnets to SI-3. In addition, the extraordinary vessel points for the indicated extraordinary vessel pair are selected and treated. In the following descriptions S^{600} indicates the aluminum and south pole combination and N^{600} indicates the gold and north pole combination.

Yin Wei Mai, Chong Mai Connection

Step 1: Determine if the left inner eye of the knee is more or less reactive than the right inner eye of the knee. Confirm by palpation between lumbar vertebrae L2 to L5.

Step 2: Choose, then treat the proper points.

Most Reactive Area	Side	Point	Metal — Magnet	Vessel
Left knee	Right	SP-4	N^{600}	chong
Left knee	Right	PC-6	S^{600}	yin wei
Left knee	Both	SI-3	N^{600}	du
Left knee	Both	BL-62	S^{600}	yang qiao
Left knee	Right	N-I	S^{600}	
Right knee	Left	SP-4	N^{600}	chong
Right knee	Left	PC-6	S^{600}	yin wei
Right knee	Both	SI-3	N^{600}	du
Right knee	Both	BL-62	S^{600}	yang qiao
Right knee	Left	N-I	S^{600}	

A patient for whom this treatment is indicated would evidence reactivity on one, not both, of the inner eyes of the knee and pressure pain between lumbar vertebrae two to five. Typical presenting symptoms are stomach or duodenal ulcer.

Yin Qiao Mai, Ren Mai Connection

Step 1: Determine that either or both of the areas on the medial side of the knees are reactive and that one or more of BL-23, BL-32, BL-33 and josen are reactive.

Step 2: Treat these points:

Most Reactive Area	Side	Point	Metal — Magnet	Vessel
Either knee	Both	KI-6	N^{600}	yin qiao
Either knee	Both	LU-7	S^{600}	ren
Either knee	Both	SI-3	N^{600}	du
Either knee	Both	BL-62	S^{600}	yang qiao
Either knee	Both	N-II	S^{600}	

A patient with stiff shoulders, cold feet and gynecological problems, pressure pain on the medial sides of both knees and pressure pain on BL-23 and BL-32 would be typical.

Yang Wei Mai, Dai Mai Connection

Step 1: Ascertain if there is a leg length difference; this is the determining factor.

Step 2: Confirm by palpating the outer eyes of the knees and the lateral and superior corners of the sacrum.

Step 3: Choose points based on the longer leg.

Longer Leg	Side	Point	Metal — Magnet	Vessel
Right	Left	TW-5	N^{600}	yang wei mai
Right	Right	GB-41	S^{600}	dai mai
Right	Both	BL-62	S^{600}	yang qiao mai
Right	Both	SI-3	N^{600}	du mai
Right	Left	P-I	N^{600}	
Left	Right	TW-5	N^{600}	yang wei mai
Left	Left	GB-41	S^{600}	dai mai
Left	Both	SI-3	N^{600}	du mai
Left	Both	BL-62	S^{600}	yang qiao mai
Left	Right	P-I	N^{600}	

The areas on the knees and sacrum are not determining factors for this treatment; these areas are diagnostically useful for checking the results of the treatment. If any reaction found in these areas has decreased, this indicates that treatment will be quickly successful.

The yang qiao and du mai pair is not commonly treated alone. It represents the axis of the body where deviations manifest as yin qiao mai and ren mai imbalances, yin wei mai and chong wei mai imbalances or yang wei mai and dai mai imbalances. The focus of treatment is on these imbalances; the yang qiao, du mai points are added to reinforce the treatments.

Note that these treatments are readily adaptable to home therapy. For chronic cases, the Ito magnets or zinc, copper and magnets may be given to the patient with the specific instructions for location and duration of treatment. Using metal balls and magnets instead of the more expensive Ito magnets is possible, but will effect a less potent stimulation.

That these treatments are able to release tension in the knees, sacrum and lower back and are able to treat leg length differences, stomach ulcers and other presenting problems is another clue to the function of the extraordinary vessels. We see how the extraordinary vessels are able to change the structural homeostasis of the body. Structural integrity is the result of complex interactions among many factors such as energetic function, muscle tension and tonicity, and fascial binding. The extraordinary vessels affect the most profound processes in the human body.

Ito Specific Treatments

In his book *Juichien De Ikayio Ga Naoru,*[14] *The Treatment of Stomach Ulcers Using Eleven Yen,* Mr. Ito offers a remarkable treatment for stomach ulcers. The reference to "Eleven Yen" is to the one yen (aluminum) and ten yen (copper) coins that may be used to treat this condition. Eight important signs evidence a stomach ulcer that is associated with the yin wei mai and chong mai. These are:

1. Bunions or other problems of the big toes or on the spleen meridians.
2. Swelling, puffiness or a knot that is painful with pressure in the knee areas previously described.
3. A noticeable pain felt in the big toe when the patient experiences fatigue.
4. A dark or purple nail color of the big toe.
5. With the patient lying face down, place your fingers on the iliac crests and press the back muscles with your thumbs at the level of your fingers. Tightness or pain indicates an ulcer. When ulcer patients are tired, a tapping massage in this area achieves comfort.
6. Pain that runs between the shoulder blades (most common with general stomach problems).
7. A flattened appearance of upper back (most common with actual stomach ulcers).
8. The area below the ribs feels tight or painful on palpation (chest distress).

If you find all or most of these signs, particularly pain around the medial eyes of the knees, you may confirm the diagnosis of a yin wei—chong mai associated stomach ulcer. Use the chong mai connection treatment. Since ulcers usually result from stress, make sure the patient is warm, relaxed and comfortable. Mr. Ito comments that the pulse should improve with this treatment. Some patients report a brief stabbing pain. This will pass. The treatment usually takes about twenty minutes; afterward, patients commonly become more alert. This treatment can be repeated as often as needed until the stomach ulcer is cured, and may be used by the patient at home.

Mr. Ito's treatment of leg length differences is similar to the yang wei mai—dai mai connection and may be used as a replacement treatment, as it is specific to leg length differences. Since this structural defect is a consequence of extant stress that has displaced the hips, it creates stress when walking. Problems of the lower and upper back, shoulders, neck and head become manifest. This imbalance should be treated first for those patients who have it. If the patient shows some of the yin qiao—ren mai signs, or if the leg length difference is clear, one inch or more, then this rather than the yang wei—dai mai treatment would generally be indicated.

Step 1: Have the patient lie on their abdomen; make sure the body is straight. Compare the leg lengths by examining the heels.

Step 2: If there is an imbalance, be sure that it is not the result of a physical difference in the length of the leg bone from surgery or accident.

Step 3: Use the following points:

Side	**Point**	**Metal — Magnet**
Longer leg	KI-6	N^{600}
Longer leg	GB-41	S^{600}
Both	BL-62	S^{600}
Both	SI-3	N^{600}
Shorter leg side	TW-5	N^{600}
Shorter leg side	LU-7	S^{600}
Shorter leg side	P-I	N^{600}
Shorter leg side	N-II	S^{600}

Make sure the patient remains warm, comfortable and relaxed. Treatment may take from five to twenty minutes, depending on the severity of the difference and the complications of the case. The legs will usually be even or closer together by the end of this treatment; sometimes you will actually watch it happen, it happens so quickly. Leg length should be checked regularly. At times a recurring difference may require a series of treatments. This treatment is also suitable for home therapy.

If the left leg is longer the problem is often easier to treat than if the right leg is longer. The following procedure is a reliable means of determining whether a leg length imbalance may be easily treated and should be done before treatment:

Step	Action
Step 1:	Place a N^{600} on the point halfway between the jing point and the crease of the finger on the external side of the middle finger P-I correspondent to the yang wei mai (on the side with the shorter leg).
Step 2:	Touch a S^{600} to the point directly opposite on the same finger N-II correspondent to the yin qiao mai for two or three seconds.
Step 3:	Check the leg lengths. If the leg lengths become equal or have shifted toward equal, this is a sign that the problem will be easy to treat. If there is no change, the problem will be more difficult to treat.

Mr. Ito tapes magnets on both P-I and N-II on the shorter leg side, retaining these, while the other N^{600} and S^{600} magnets are taped on the body.

Occasionally, the difference in leg length is not clear. With such a case, do not test the middle finger; you could adjust the patient's legs the wrong way. Instead, have the patient slowly turn their head to the left, then to the right. If there is an imbalance, the leg you suspect to be shorter will move or become clearly shorter.

If these treatments do not correct the leg length, palpate the area slightly superior to the midpoint on a line between GB-20 and GB-12 on the side of the shorter leg. Usually, you will find some slight tension, a knot or pain. Palpate gently and quickly; do not overpalpate or palpate the longer leg side. Find the most reactive point and use moxa. Mr. Ito also recommends the use of a laser to stimulate this point for a few seconds. If the pain and tension at this point decreases, the reactive area on the knee will change; the sterno-cleidomastoid muscle will become looser and the leg length difference should decrease. In these cases, where the moxa or laser treatment is necessary, the leg length problem will be found to be the result of a first or second cervical vertebrae displacement complicating the yang wei mai imbalance.

Ito Adjunctive Magnetic Therapy

There are many ways of using magnets, electric fields and currents.[15] These techniques may be used as complete treatments, as Ms. Tokito does, or as the preparation for local treatments or in combination with other treatments. While the combinations of extraordinary vessel therapy with local treatments are potentially as various as imaginative practitioners may wish to make them, the two basic methods used by Mr. Ito have given encouraging results and aptly demonstrate the method of combination. With the first method, Mr. Ito focusses on the reactive knee and lower back areas. If both are reactive, he will treat both. For example, someone suffering from sciatica who has a longer left leg, left lateral knee reactivity and tenderness at the left superior lateral corner of the sacrum would receive the following treatment:

Side	Point	Metal — Magnet
Both	SI-3	N^{600} (600 gauss)
Right	TW-5	N^{600} (600 gauss)
Both	BL-62	S^{600} (600 gauss)
Left	GB-41	S^{600} (600 gauss)
Right	P-I	N^{600} (600 gauss)
Sacrum	Reactive area	$(N)^{-3000}$ (3000 gauss)
Knee	Reactive area	$(S)^{-3000}$ (3000 gauss)

The 3000 gauss magnets would be attached to the pointer machine and stimulated electrically. This reinforces the extraordinary vessel treatment, allowing for greater structural adjustment and greater stimulation of energetic blockages and, thereby, reinforcing the root treatment. In this instance the treatment of SI-3, TW-5, BL-62 and GB-41 are the standard root treatment. Treatment of the reactive sacral and knee areas is included because it works on the root diagnostic reflex areas and supports the root treatment, encouraging rapid change by unblocking the energies at the pivotal reflex areas.

If one, but not both of the knee or sacral reflex areas are found to be particularly reactive, the treatment can be applied in two ways. Either place the magnets as described, though reactivity was found in only one area, or place the (N)$^{-3000}$ on the reactive area and the (S)$^{-3000}$ approximately two to three centimeters below. If this does not produce a reduction in reactivity, try placing the (S)$^{-3000}$ on another distal point. For instance, for a reaction in the yang wei knee area, placing (N)$^{-3000}$ on the reactive area and a (S)$^{-3000}$ on GB-34 is often helpful.

The polarity and placement of the magnets to be stimulated electrically is dependent on the patient's complaints and the areas of reactivity. If the first patient, with reaction on both the knee and sacrum, evidenced lower back, neck or shoulder pain, the polarity and placement may have been the same — the area of the local problem is similar. However, if the patient's complaint had been knee pain, the polarity would have been reversed. The (N)$^{-3000}$ would have been placed at the reactive knee area and the (S)$^{-3000}$ at the reactive sacral area. The (N)$^{-3000}$ is placed on the painful area. While we do not speak of tonification or sedation when using magnetic therapy, the (N)$^{-3000}$ effects may be thought of as a parallel to dispersion and the (S)$^{-3000}$ effects as a parallel to tonification. For example, with knee pain in the yin wei mai—chong mai reactive areas, the (N)$^{-3000}$ could be placed on the reactive knee area and the (S)$^{-3000}$ on a point slightly medial to HT-7 on the same side. Mr. Ito reports he has successfully treated over two thousand patients with knee problems using these combinations and applying the principles previously described. The same combination is effective in treating intercostal neuralgia and heart problems.

He has found several other point combinations effective for reactiveness in the diagnostic reflex areas.[16] For a patient with a yin qiao mai problem and strong pressure pain on josen, use the following: N^{600} to SI-3, KI-6 bilaterally, and S^{600} to BL-62, S^{600} to LU-7 bilaterally, (N)$^{-3000}$ either side of the sore josen point and a corresponding (S)$^{-3000}$ on GB-34, left to left, right to right.

Side	Point	Metal-Magnet
Both	KI-6	N^{600}
Both	SI-3	N^{600}
Both	LU-7	S^{600}
Both	BL-62	S^{600}
Both	N-II	S^{600}
Left of	Josen	$(N)^{-3000}$
Left	GB-34	$(S)^{-3000}$
Right of	Josen	$(N)^{-3000}$
Right	GB-34	$(S)^{-3000}$

For a yin qiao mai diagnosis with tightness at BL-23 and other kidney symptoms, as well as treating SI-3, KI-6, BL-62 and LU-7, place a $(N)^{-3000}$ on each reactive BL-23 and the $(S)^{-3000}$ on a point near BL-53 on the lateral edges of the popliteal crease.

Side	Point	Metal-Magnet
Both	KI-6	N^{600}
Both	SI-3	N^{600}
Both	LU-7	S^{600}
Both	BL-62	S^{600}
Both	N-II	S^{600}
Left	BL-23	$(N)^{-3000}$
Left	around BL-53	$(S)^{-3000}$
Right	BL-23	$(N)^{-3000}$
Right	around BL-53	$(S)^{-3000}$

For a badly strained back centered around the L4 to L5 joint, treat N^{600} SI-3, SP-4 bilaterally and S^{600} BL-62, PC-6 bilaterally with four $(N)^{-3000}$ placed around the L4-L5 joint as follows. The corresponding $(S)^{-3000}$ should be connected on the same sides to GB-34 and the reactive knee yin wei areas:

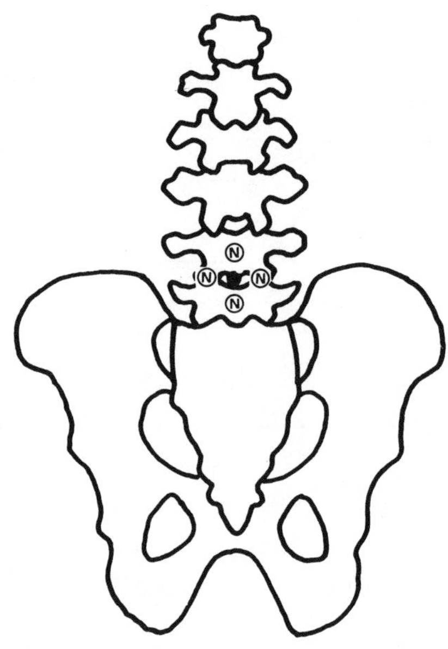

Figure 34

Side	Point	Metal-Magnet
Both	SP-4	N^{600}
Both	SI-3	N^{600}
Both	PC-6	S^{600}
Both	BL-62	S^{600}
Both	N-I	S^{600}
around	lumbar 4-5	$(N)^{-3000}$ X 4
Both	GB-34	$(S)^{-3000}$
Both	reactive knee areas	$(S)^{-3000}$

In a stomach ulcer, as well as the regular Ito magnet treatment, if the area around left ST-21 is reactive, one can place $(N)^{-3000}$ on ST-21 and $(S)^{-3000}$ on the reactive knee yin wei area.

Side	Point	Metal-Magnet
Both	SI-3	N^{600}
Right	SP-4	N^{600}
Both	BL-62	S^{600}
Right	PC-6	S^{600}
Right	N-I	S^{600}
Left	ST-21	$(N)^{-3000}$
Left	reactive knee area	$(S)^{-3000}$

The second adjunctive style of treatment recommended by Mr. Ito focusses on the area of the problem: the most painful point, or a very reactive point associated with the condition. There are numerous principles that may be applied. Many of these principles stem from classical sources; some are derived from the work of Tsugio Nagatomo[17] and Dr. Yoshio Manaka[18] as well as the work of Mr. Ito.[19] These principles are:

1. Treat the reactive area directly with the $(N)^{-3000}$ and a point reflecting that area with the $(S)^{-3000}$.

2. Treat the reactive area according to a left—right balance.

3. Treat the reactive area with the $(N)^{-3000}$ and use the $(S)^{-3000}$ further downstream on the same meridian to drain the reactive area.

As an example of the first principle, consider a patient with shoulder problems and a yang wei mai imbalance. Treat the extraordinary vessels with the Ito magnets and treat GB-21 with $(N)^{-3000}$ and LI-10 with $(S)^{-3000}$, if there is pressure pain on both of these points. LI-10 has a well-known effect on shoulder pain and tension. Similarly, for shoulder pain, treating a palpable vein above the clavicle (roughly in the center of the clavicle) with $(N)^{-3000}$, and LU-8 on the same side with $(S)^{-3000}$, can be effective. We can summarize this treatment in the following table:

Side	**Point**	**Metal-Magnet**
Both	SI-3	N^{600}
Both	BL-62	S^{600}
Right	TW-5	N^{600}
Left	GB-41	S^{600}
Right	P-I	N^{600}
Both	GB-21	$(N)^{-3000}$
Both	LI-10	$(S)^{-3000}$
Both	Vein above clavicle	$(N)^{-3000}$
Both	LU-8	$(S)^{-3000}$

A patient with headache and a yin qiao mai—ren mai imbalance could be treated by combining the extraordinary vessel treatment and Ito magnets. Place (N)$^{-3000}$ on GB-20 and (S)$^{-3000}$ on LI-4 or on the backache—neck tension point on the back of the hand, located on the dorsal side of the junction of the fourth and fifth metacarpals. Choose the sore point. This treatment is summarized as follows:

Side	Point	Metal-Magnet
Both	LU-7	S^{600}
Both	KI-6	N^{600}
Both	SI-3	N^{600}
Both	BL-62	S^{600}
Both	N-II	S^{600}
Both	GB-20	(N)$^{-3000}$
Both	LI-4 or hand neck point	(S)$^{-3000}$

Arthritic pain is a good example of the use of the second and third principles. Consider, for example, arthritic pain around LI-4.[20] If the pain is one sided, we can apply the second principle, what Akabane called the "see-saw phenomenon."[21] If left LI-4 is arthritic, right LI-4 will also be affected, but in an opposite way. Pain generally indicates an excess; thus, left LI-4 is relatively excess and right LI-4 is relatively deficient. For a simple treatment we may place a north magnet on left LI-4 and a south magnet on right LI-4. Often this alone is a sufficient treatment for arthritic pain. However, if this doesn't work, or if the pain is bilateral, we need to apply the third principle.

Placing north "upstream" on the most reactive point and south "downstream" at a point further from the beginning of the meridian often relieves pain. In the example case, if left LI-4 is sore, place the (N)$^{-3000}$ on left LI-4. Then, palpate roughly four to five centimeters down the meridian, between LI-5 and LI-6 for example, and find a reactive point. Place the (S)$^{-3000}$ here. This treatment works by encouraging the excess, where the pain is, to flow down the meridian, like clearing a blockage in a stream of water. This treatment may be bilateral if necessary.

For simple arthritic conditions, one of these two treatment principles will suffice. More complicated cases require other principles of operation. Another approach uses the north magnet to disperse the excess at the painful point; the south pole is used to tonify a related point or area where there is a relative deficiency. Assume that in addition to arthritis of the left hand around LI-4, or a yin wei—chong mai disharmony with reaction on the left knee area, there is an accompanying deficient liver, spleen or kidney condition. In such a condition, we can use the south magnet to tonify the deficiency. For instance, when there is a deficient kidney condition, place the south magnet on a point that will tonify the deficient kidney.

Selecting the point for placement of the (N)-3000 is simple; however, selection of the point to receive the (S)-3000 is tricky. It is necessary that the point chosen provide the potential connection whereby the differences in polarity between the (N)-3000 and the (S)-3000 may link. It is not only necessary that this linking occur; it is necessary that the currents thus established are stimulating an appropriate energetic relationship. In this regard, magnetic therapy and needle acupuncture share an identical principle. If we imagine the body as a sphere, the person's pain or complaint may be seen as a bump on the surface of this sphere. Every bump will have an accompanying depression somewhere on the surface.

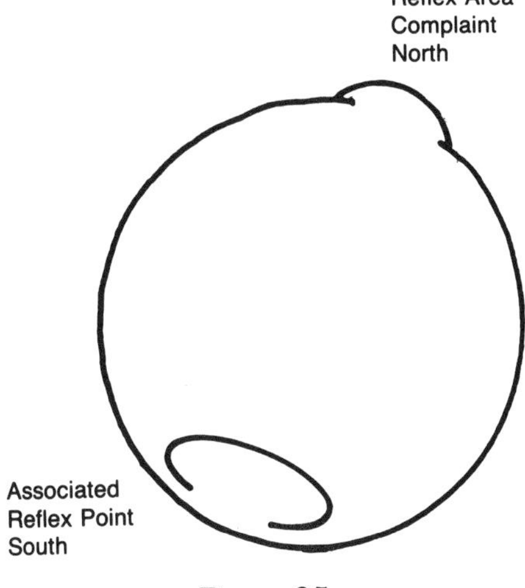

Figure 35

The (N)-3000 will be placed either on the bump or a point that is strongly related; the (S)-3000 will be placed either on the depression or a strongly related point. The bumps are usually easy to find, since the patient tells us their complaints. The depressions are harder to locate and generally not so visible. In effect, we are searching for the point that will create the gradient necessary for the currents to work effectively when associated with the painful point. In the preceding examples this association has been made by the location of the local problem or through the association of reflex areas. However, it will be necessary or desirable to use other principles.

The location of the corresponding point is complicated by the fact that the human body does not have as symmetrical a shape as our imaginary sphere. Also, there may be more than one depression. The depression results from a variety of causes and may be located anywhere on the surface. All the diagnostic models may be used to determine where we locate the point to use in association with the painful point, for each concerns the body's balance and energetic structure. Since we can not always find the critical depression in one try, a systematic and iterative process is required.

We recommend beginning with Mr. Ito's treatment style. If the results are not satisfying, use your treatment logic to determine the appropriate point to associate with the extraordinary vessel treatment. In our experience there are three combination systems that have provided excellent results:

- treating scars
- tonifying deficient element conditions
- treating zones described by Dr. Zhang Xin Shu of China.

While each of these three combination systems could be used as a complete therapy, our experience combining these with Mr. Ito's style of practice encourages us to recommend the combination method. For his treatments of the extraordinary vessels, a pointer machine is used to stimulate the magnets on the relevant points. Use of this technique is again presumed in the following examples.

Scar Treatments

Treating scars is really a special case of using the Ito method; the scar is treated as a local problem when there are indications that it is energetically pathological.[22] Most often, pathological scars are on or across a meridian. Signs of pathology include patient complaints of discomfort, recurring pain or pressure pain. For example, you may find sharp pressure pain on one or more points along the scar or a feeling of discomfort that radiates when pressed. These reactive points are the points treated. Place the (N)$^{-3000}$ on the most reactive point and the (S)$^{-3000}$ further down the meridian on the scar or on a reactive point downstream on the meridian. The most effective point may be as close as one to three inches or as far as the end of the meridian. Assume, for example, a patient with left knee pain who has already had surgery on the knee. The pain and scar are both in the reactive yin wei mai—chong mai reflex area. The scar is sore to the touch. One would treat:

Side	Point	Metal-Magnet
Right	PC-6	S^{600}
Right	SP-4	N^{600}
Both	SI-3	N^{600}
Both	BL-62	S^{600}
Right	N-I	S^{600}
Left	Sore scar point	(N)$^{-3000}$
Left	Medial to HT-7	(S)$^{-3000}$

Should this combination prove unsuccessful after five to ten minutes of treatment, the (S)$^{-3000}$ could be moved to a sore point on the scar, if one can be found. If this does not eliminate the pressure pain on the scar, or if there is no second point on or just below the scar, palpate further up the meridian, around SP-10 or higher, and select a point.

Five Element Deficiency Treatments

In the element and stem or five element treatment styles, deficient element diagnoses are frequent. Treatment of these deficiencies are productively combined with extraordinary vessel treatments. To create combination treatments a clear diagnosis is necessary. You must determine that the problem is single or multi-element and select the single point best suited to the condition. Single element imbalances are simpler. According to the *Nan Jing* they are also easier to treat. In cases where more than one element is involved, it is necessary to determine if the elements are transforming through the creative or controlling cycle.

In single meridian problems, such as a deficient spleen, tonify the spleen meridian by tonifying SP-3 or SP-4, depending on which is more reactive. Based on the reports of many modern Japanese practitioners, these have been found to be more effective than SP-2. Alternately, you might tonify the horary point of the mother meridian, PC-8. Since use of the (S)-3000 is the parallel of tonification in the five element model, the (S)-3000 is used to treat the points requiring tonification. Thus, for a patient who evidenced yin wei mai—chong mai reactivity, diagnosed as having an uncomplex spleen deficiency, the (N)-3000 would be placed on the reactive knee area and the (S)-3000 on SP-3, SP-4 or PC-8. Similarly, LU-9 would receive the (S)-3000 for lung deficiency. If the results are not satisfactory, use SP-3. LU-6 may be a useful point, if it is reactive. It is used for acute conditions, as are accumulation points in general. Our experience shows that LU-6 is sometimes effective for chronic deficiencies. Thus, someone with a yin qiao mai—ren mai problem, with lung deficiency, pressure pain on the inside of the left knee and pressure pain on right LU-9, treatment would consist of placing the (N)-3000 on the left knee and (S)-3000 on right LU-9. On occasion, LU-7 may also be used with the (S)-3000. Luo points can be good for tonification.

In liver deficiency, LV-8 or LV-3 may be selected, as may KI-10. In kidney deficiency KI-7 is usually treated, but KI-3 may also be helpful. If neither work, apply the (S)-3000 to LU-8. Problems of the heart are excess problems. Some practitioners feel that it is inappropriate to treat the heart meridian because the heart is the "emperor" and stores the shen. For heart problems, palpate the pericardium meridian. Generally, either PC-4 or PC-6 will be sore; treat the reactive point.

For two meridian problems associated by the creative cycle, such as liver and kidney deficiency, tonify the horary point of the mother meridian, KI-10. Similarly, for creative cycle spleen and lung deficiency, tonify SP-3. To treat two meridians that relate on the controlling cycle, such as a liver and spleen deficiency, begin by tonifying one meridian. To do so, first determine the most affected of the two meridians, then tonify its horary or tonification point. In this example, we would tonify LV-1 or LV-8, SP-3 or SP-2, depending on which meridian was most deficient. Sometimes it is difficult differentiating the more deficient meridian. In such cases, it is safest to treat neither. Apply some other principle. You should be able to find a pattern that fits one diagnosis well. Treat the point indicated remembering that the (N)-3000 is placed at the site of the local problem or reactive knee or sacral area. After applying the treatment of choice, examine the deficient elements again. Often the case will be clearer.

Do not treat points bilaterally; try to select an appropriate side. For instance, since the liver tends to cause problems of the left leg and since liver problems tend to be reflected by points on the left leg, treat the most reactive liver point on the left side. For lung deficiency, the right side is usually most appropriate. Heart problems tend to reflect on the left side. Problems of the other meridians are less clearly predictable. In these cases look to the pattern of abdominal reaction for clues and compare the points to be treated for reactivity. Select the side that shows greater reaction.

All the five element diagnoses and treatments are used with the reactive knee, lower back, or painful areas. For example, a case presenting:

- gynecological problems
- reaction on the yin qiao mai, ren mai knee area of both legs
- reaction on BL-32
- an element diagnosis of single meridian kidney deficiency
- reaction on CV-4, KI-7

would be treated by:

Side	Point	Metal — Magnet
Both	SI-3	N^{600}
Both	KI-6	N^{600}
Both	BL-62	S^{600}
Both	LU-7	S^{600}
Both	N-II	S^{600}
Reactive	knee yin qiao area	$(N)^{-3000}$
Reactive	KI-7	$(S)^{-3000}$

The $(S)^{-3000}$ also could have been placed on KI-3 or KI-10 on the reactive side. In this example, KI-7 was most reactive and was thus selected. If this treatment proved ineffective, the $(N)^{-3000}$ could be placed on CV-4, a reactive point on the abdomen associated with the problem. The (S)-3000 would then be placed on one of the kidney points. Though many combinations are possible for each case, if the treatment logic is clear, the results will be encouraging.

Treatments with the Zones of Dr. Zhang Xin Shu

Almost any treatment system can be combined with extraordinary vessel treatments; even individual and specialized treatment systems may be used. Since the primary effort is to locate the point or area that is energetically related to the problem targeted for treatment, many systems will work well. One system that has provided excellent results utilizes the ideas and treatment points of Dr. Zhang Xin Shu, as found in his book, *Wan Ke Zhen, Wrist Ankle Acupuncture.*[23] Dr. Zhang discovered six points above each wrist and ankle that are associated with zones on the body. Each zone is coupled with an upper and a lower treatment point. The upper points are located two finger widths above the wrist crease; the lower points are located three finger widths above the tip of the ankles:

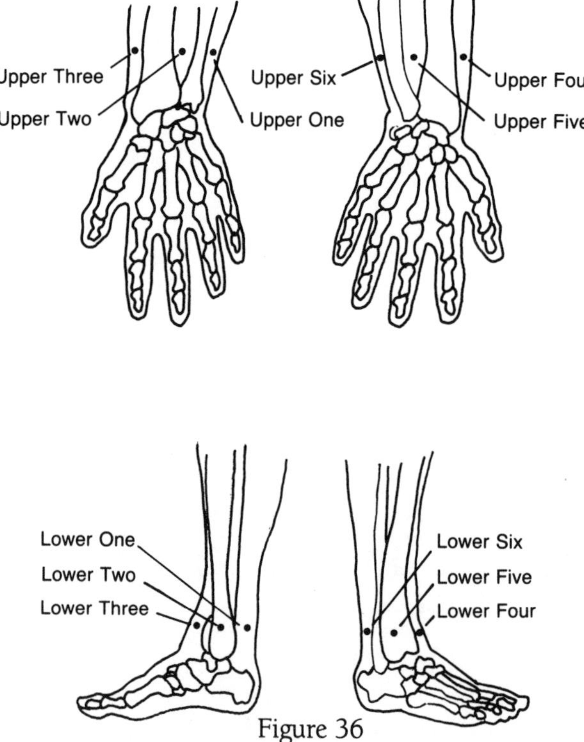

Figure 36

Zhang Xin Shu Zones — Front of Body

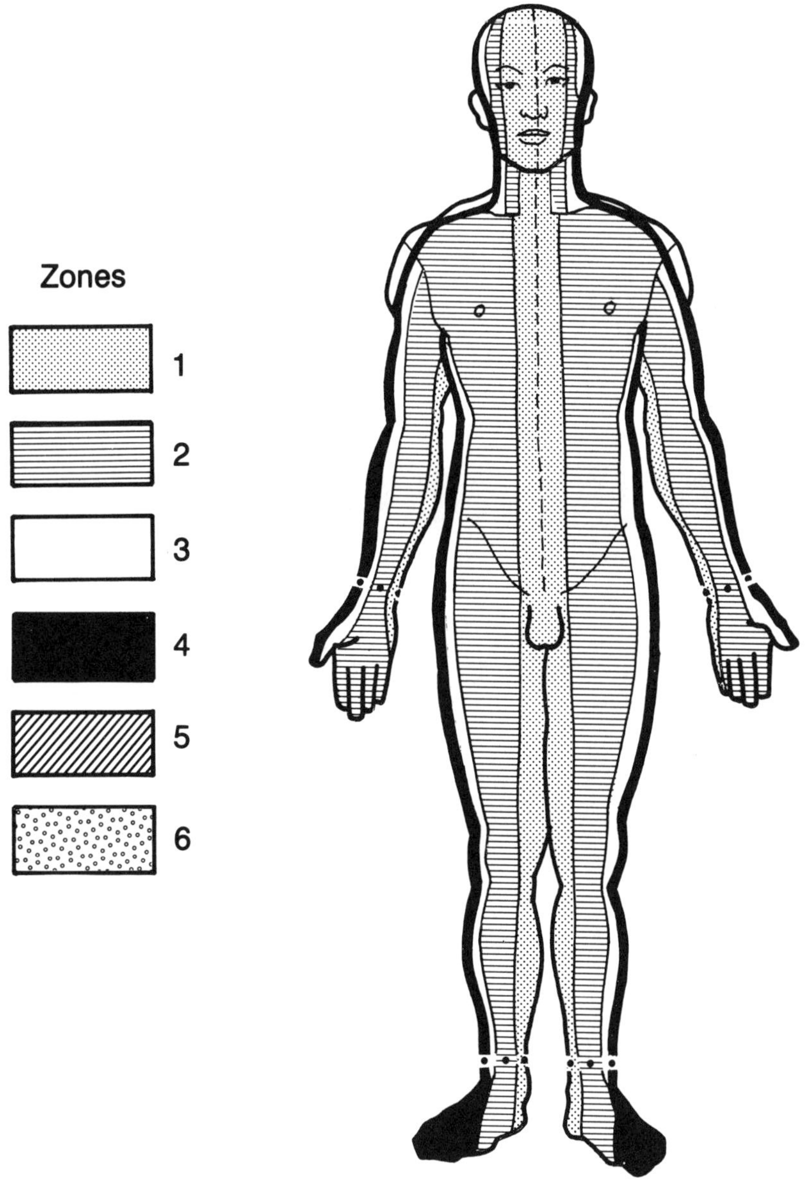

Figure 37

Zhang Xin Shu Zones — Back of Body

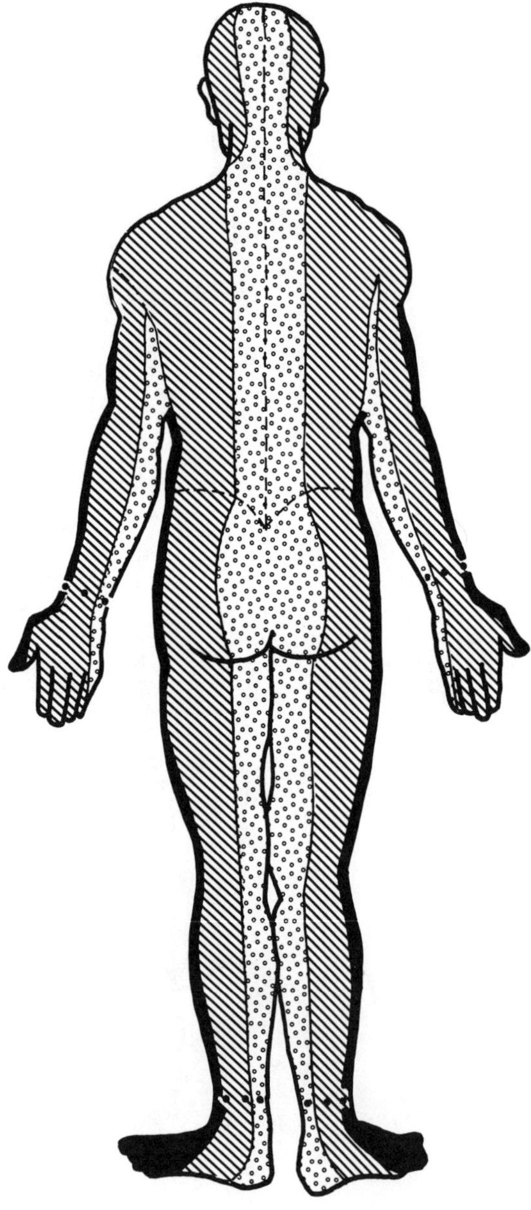

Figure 38

Zhang Xin Shu Zones — Side of Body

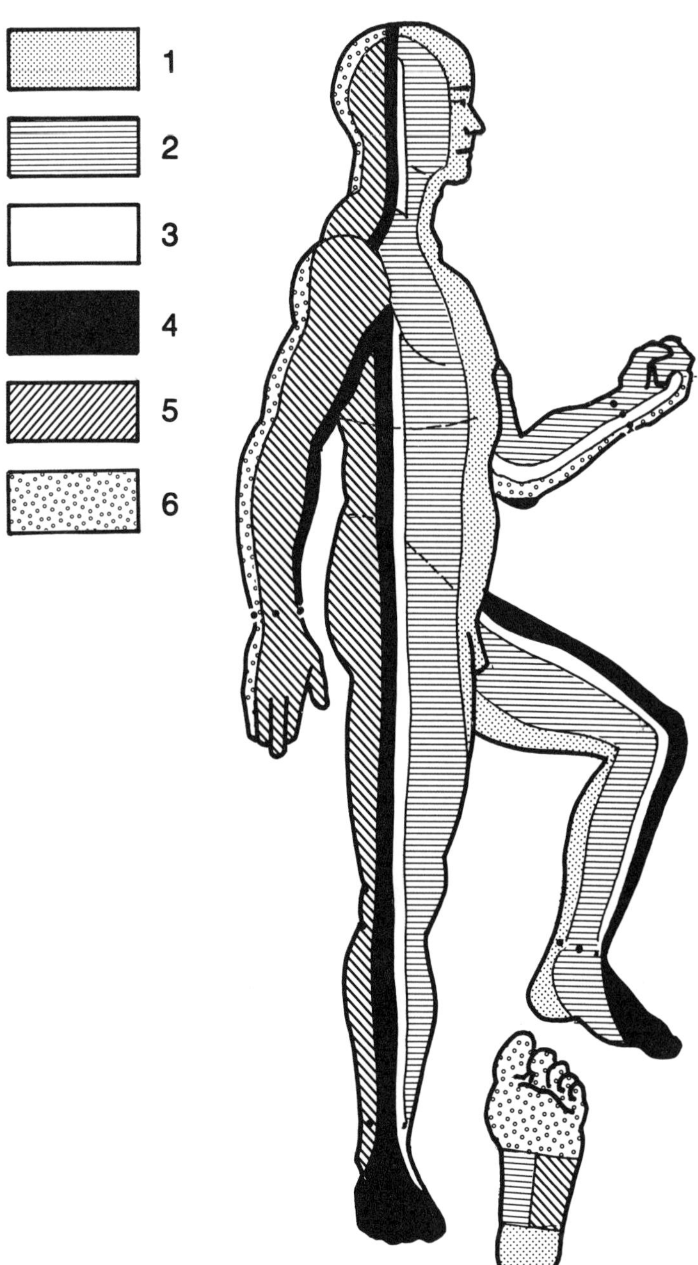

Figure 39

The six zones are roughly analagous to the coupled meridians – shao yin, tai yin, jue yin, shao yang, tai yang, yang ming. The upper points control correspondent zones above the diaphragm, the lower points control the zones below the diaphragm. However, sometimes the area between the navel and diaphragm may be reflective of the upper or lower points.

Dr. Shu has found a series of symptoms associated with each of these zones:

Upper 1:

- headache (forehead)
- irritation of the eyelids (sand in the eyes)
- declining eyesight
- chronic stuffed nose
- trigeminal neuralgia
- frontal toothache
- pharyngitis
- tonsillitis
- bronchitis
- nausea
- vomiting
- belching
- angina pectoris
- high blood pressure
- hemiplegia (affected side)
- itchiness of the whole body
- dizziness
- insomnia
- spontaneous sweating
- uncontrolled shaking
- mental disorders (hysteria, etc.)
- whole body symptoms.

Upper 2:

- headache (side)
- toothache (back)
- jaw pain
- chest pain
- asthma.

Upper 3:

- high blood pressure
- pain in the sides of the chest.

Upper 4:

- headache (top of the head)
- tinnitus
- difficulty hearing
- shoulder problems (of the front)
- pain in the sides of the chest.

Upper 5:

- headache (back)
- shoulder problems (of the back)
- numbness or oversensitivity of the upper arm
- arthritis (elbow).

Upper 6:

- headache (back)
- pain in the back of the neck.

Lower 1:

- stomachache
- pain around CV-8
- menstrual cramps
- gynecologic problems
- itchiness of the sexual organs.

Lower 2:

- pain in the liver area
- pain in the sides of the abdomen
- colitis.

Lower 3:

- knee pain (in the yin wei—chong mai diagnosis area).

Lower 4:

- pain in the thigh
- knee pain (in the yang wei—dai mai diagnosis area)
- numbness or oversensitivity of the limb.

Lower 5:

- hip joint pain.

Lower 6:

- backache
- tiredness in the lower back
- sciatica
- pain around the lateral edges of the sacrum (yang wei—dai mai diagnosis area.

He treats the correspondent points with a gentle lateral needle insertion that places the needle subcutaneously one to one and a half inches. (If the same points are treated with local treatments or treatments of reactive knee and lower back areas, use of magnets is recommended.)

Points are selected according to two principles. If the patient's problem clearly lies on a zone, above or below the diaphragm, the appropriate upper or lower point should be palpated. If it is reactive, it may be used. If the presenting symptoms are associated with one of the zones, palpate the treatment point for reaction. If the point is not reactive, the treatment is inappropriate.

Combination treatments using these points can be helpful in the treatment of stubborn knee or sacral area problems. For example, a patient with a yang wei mai—dai mai diagnosis, left leg longer, right knee yang wei mai—dai mai area reactive, with symptoms of stiff shoulders, occasional sciatica down the right gallbladder meridian, discomfort of the sacrum with palpable distress along the lateral edges of the sacrum, treatment could be:

Side	Point	Metal — Magnet
Both	SI-3	N^{600}
Right	TW-5	N^{600}
Both	BL-62	S^{600}
Left	GB-41	S^{600}
Right	P-I	N^{600}
Right	reactive knee yang wei mai area	$(N)^{-3000}$
Right	lower 6	$(S)^{-3000}$

If the selection logic is correct, favorable results might be achieved in ten to fifteen minutes.

Summary

The extraordinary vessel treatments described in this chapter fall into two basic categories: those based on the finding and differentiation of obvious left—right chi pulse imbalances, and those based on leg length differences and obvious, palpable reactions around the knees and lower back. With the first treatment style, if diagnosis and point location are accurate, nothing else is required. For the second set of treatments, depending on the severity, stubbornness and complexity of the problem, other points may be used. If you use other points, begin by working on the reactive knee and lower back areas. If the results achieved are not sufficient, determine if there are obvious five element deficiencies or if there is a body zone implicated. If neither of these is evident, a local treatment of the patient's problem should be appropriate.

The first set of treatments exemplify treatment of the deepest energetics of the extraordinary vessels described by the classics. The second set of treatments exemplify treatment of the structural relationships of the extraordinary vessels. As with the classical treatments, these are practical means of applying the principle of root treatment. Both the classical and modern treatment systems imply that the concept of gradients is worthy of further research and therapeutic consideration. Clearly, the extraordinary vessels offer an excellent means of affecting the deepest energetics of the human body.

Notes

[1] Information on Ms. Tokito's treatments is derived from lectures she gave in Tokyo in the summer of 1984.

[2] Information about Mr. Ito's treatments is reported from the author's studies with Mr. Ito in Tokyo in 1983 and 1984. Further information has been taken from his book, *Juichien de Ikayio ga Naoru,* the *Treatment of Stomach Ulcers Using Eleven Yen,* from his seminars and from his seminar handbook, *Magnetic Electric Acupuncture Without Needles, PIA Therapy.* Mr. Ito is currently writing his own English language book that covers his treatment style and techniques.

[3] *Zhen Jiu Da Cheng,* p. 182.

[4] Mr. Nagatomo makes extensive reference to Bachmann's work in his *Nagatomo M.P. Shinkyu Kuowa Hachiju Hachisyu.*

[5] The chart is derived from Osamu Ito, *Juichien de Ikayio ga Naoru,* p. 68.

[6] See *Hara: Reflections on the Sea.*

[7] See "Magnetic field deficiency syndrome and magnetic treatment," *Japan Medical Journal,* No. 2745, Dec. 1976.

[8] *Nan Jing,* Chapter 18. See also, *Five Elements and Ten Stems,* pp. 113-115 *passim.*

[9] *Nan Jing,* Chapter 8.

[10] In *Su Wen,* Chapter 21, there is a reference to the "pivot" nature of the kidneys.

[11] Described in *Hara: Reflections on the Sea.*

[12] Mr. Ito's book, *Juichien de Ikayio ga Naoru,* concentrates on the treatment of stomach ulcers for the lay person and the professional. He is famous for his results with this disease, though he has good results treating knee pain as well.

[13] See further, *Lectures on KoRyo SooJi Chim, Korean Hand Acupuncture.* Seoul: Eum Yang Maek Jin Publishing Co., 1976.

[14] Osamu Ito, *Juichien de Ikayio ga Naoru*, p. 44.

[15] Dr. Yoshio Manaka uses them frequently in his treatments. See *Hara: Reflections on the Sea*. Dr. Chen Zhi of the Hunan province in China uses them exclusively. See his *Ci Liao Fa, Magnet Therapy*.

[16] Described in Mr. Ito's seminars and seminar handbook, *Magnetic Electric Acupuncture Without Needles*.

[17] Nagatomo, *Nagatomo M.P. Shinkyu Kuowa Hachiju Hachisyu*.

[18] Dr. Manaka demonstrates these ideas in his clinic and lectures and references them occasionally in his many books.

[19] *Ibid.*

[20] The information concerning arthritic pain around LI-4 comes from *Nagatomo M.P. Shinkyu Kuowa Hachiju Hachisyu*, and from private discussions with the author.

[21] See K. Akabane, *Hinaishin Ho*, p. 16. A similar idea can be found in the *Su Wen*, Chapter 27.

[22] Dr. Chen Zhi reports good success with patients by treating reactive scars.

[23] *Wan Ke Zhen, Wrist Ankle Acupuncture*. Translated into Japanese by Mitsutane Sugi and published by Ido no Nippon Sha, 1979.

Extraordinary Vessels

Extraordinary Vessel Points Actions and Effects

The actions and effects of extraordinary vessel points are a more difficult research question than the actions of meridian points. Since the points are most often used in combination, an extraordinary vessel action is specifically described only where the master–coupled pair are clearly given as the effective stimulus. How the classical authors thought of the master and coupled points of the extraordinary vessels is fairly clear. At least, when they thought that the points were acting through the extraordinary vessels, they indicated that this was the case. However, these points are also meridian points, each having an individual "reputation" as such. For standardized textbooks the actions of each point are, more or less, the sum of the agreements among authors at the time the text was composed, the basics for which there is general accord. In more specialized books the effects are those that either an individual practitioner or school of practitioners considers important.

Distinction between a point acting as an extraordinary vessel stimulus and the same point acting as a meridian stimulus is not necessarily clear. The only certain distinction must be derived by theorizing, testing and measuring. We must ask and answer at least three questions:

> 1. *Is an extraordinary vessel action involved only when both the master and coupled point pair is stimulated?*
>
> 2. *Is the stimulation of the extraordinary vessel points by some specific type of stimulation the key that determines if an extraordinary vessel action will be induced?*
>
> 3. *Do the body's energies respond to the stimulation of an extraordinary vessel point through the extraordinary vessels only when there is a related imbalance?*

The measurements that would be required to answer these questions have not been done and may not even be possible with current tools. Each practitioner who has used the extraordinary vessels extensively has operated from a theory, and clearly the ideas of fields, gradients and biases that have inspired the modern techniques may claim considerable objective success by their results.

These questions are interesting and each of the theoretical answers we might suggest will produce further questions. If, for example, we debate that any stimulus of these points, by any means, will involve both meridian and extraordinary vessel changes, what part of the reputation of each of these points is really due to the function of the extraordinary vessel involved? Practically, however, these questions cannot be answered immediately, nor are the answers necessary to make use of the information. We can use a guide that permits us to make informed treatment selections. In this regard, comparison of point effects gives us a reasonable beginning and makes an interesting study. As a beginning, we have included the point indication descriptions provided by the modern Chinese textbook, *Zhen Jiu Xue*.[1]

These descriptions serve as a basis for the point as "meridian point" indication comparisons. An obvious comparative selection would have been a modern Chinese discussion of the treatment points as master and coupled point pairs. However, we did not find much distinctive discussion of the extraordinary vessels in the available modern literature. The one book we did find, the *Zi Wu Zhen Jiu Liao Fa*, gave the *Ju Ying* and *Da Cheng* indications for each of the eight points, with no further modern discussion. The one extraordinary vessel text in English that would appear to represent modern Chinese practice[2] is completely without therapeutic principles or source references.

Two modern practitioners who have made the appropriate distinctions, and who have complete lists of point indications for the eight extraordinary vessel points, are Tsugio Nagatomo, the father of the "minus—plus" acupuncture system, and Gerhard Bachmann, the German acupuncturist who introduced the concept to him.[3] Because they have also compiled symptomologies for the extraordinary vessels, we have chosen to feature their work as a good comparison to the meridian point work from the *Zhen Jiu Xue*.

To make the comparison wider and easier to use, we have assembled for each of the eight vessels a collation of the indications for the corresponding master and coupled points. This amounts to an informal statistical analysis of the point effects. In addition to the modern and classical sources detailed in the text, there are two other sources considered: *Acupuncture a Comprehensive Text* and the *Book of Acupuncture Points* by James Tin-Yau So. These provide, respectively, information from another modern standard text (Shanghai) and the personal experience of a respected practitioner from a line of well-known teachers.

A number of points must be kept in mind. First, the collation of point effects has required some abbreviation, simply to fit the format. While the sections for each extraordinary vessel do provide a handy repertoire, the symptoms and associated point lists are incomplete for a few of the entries. The lists of points for the classical point combinations have been replaced with the abbreviation "CC." Since the texts used span several centuries, the differences in language and presentation have required some compromise. The modern texts tend to use disease names where convenient, the older texts use symptom and sign sets. The multiple comparison sections are organized by body area to include, as much as possible, similar problems within the same grouping. A more liberal interpretation could have included more of the symptoms in some of the groups. Finally, in any precise sense, the fact that a variety of sources agree on the indications for a particular point "proves" nothing. Certainly, an accord that a point affects a particular problem strongly suggests its use. Where the experience of those sources that have used the extraordinary vessels is in accord, we may assume a clinical rule. Where the sources that concentrate on meridian point effects differ from the sources that specify extraordinary vessel effects, we can posit that an actual energetic distinction is likely. However, strong words such as "proof" are not in order.

Zhen Jiu Xue Indications

Point	Indications
SP-4	stomachache; vomiting; indigestion; abdominal pain; diarrhea; diseases that cause diarrhea
PC-6	angina; heart palpitations; stomachache; nausea and vomiting; madness; epilepsy; heat diseases; spasming pain of the elbows and arms
LU-7	cough; panting; chest pain; hand or arm pain; sore throat
KI-6	irregular menses; red or white discharge; itchy genitals; frequent urination; constipation; beri-beri; swollen legs; epilepsy; insomnia; difficulty passing urine

GB-41 pain at the lateral canthus of the eye; rib cage painful; irregular menses; dripping urine; swelling and pain of the dorsum of the feet; spasming pain of the toes

TW-5 heat diseases; headache; deafness; tinnitus; red, swollen, painful eyes; rib cage pain; difficulty bending, stretching arm and elbow; sharp pain of the hands and fingers

SI-3 heat diseases with no sweat; headache; shoulder, upper arm, neck pain; finger spasms; wrist pain; jaundice

BL-62 epilepsy; madness; headache; dizziness; sharp pain of the back and thigh

Nagatomo and Bachmann Meridian Point Indications

Point **Indications**

SP-4: heart and circulatory problems; heart pain; angina; heart palpitations; heat that causes suffering in the heart; pressure in the chest; conjunctivitis; no appetite; constant yawning; heartburn; liver diseases; hemorrhoid pain; anal prolapse; varicose veins; difficulty with menstruation; cystitis; late labor {often a chong mai problem}; rheumatic problems, particularly of the muscles and joints; spasming of the eyelid; tinnitus; whole body spasms; stomach spasms; intestinal spasms; rapid palpitations; catarrh of the stomach or intestines; stomach ulcer; gallstone pain; pancreatitis; sharp pain in the back; constipation; difficulty urinating; stiffness of the penis

PC-6: congestion of the brain; heart pain; pericarditis and carditis; hepatitis; hemorrhoids; hot diseases; arthritis of the elbow; hand spasms; phobias; amnesia; weakness; allergies; catarrh of the intestines; melancholia; borborygmus; lack of sexual satisfaction during sex; yawning; gingivitis; night blindness; herniated intestines; blood pressure problems; impotence; nervous breakdown; nephritis; inflammation in the mouth; lazy eye; dizziness.

LU-7: diseases of the body mucosa; stagnation of the respiratory system or lower abdomen in women (menstrual problems, unusual menses, discharge); stagnation in the lower abdomen that is related to stagnation in the head {for instance, gynecologic problems causing problems in the head}; acne; skin problems that cause peeling of the skin; lipomas; insufficient lactation; problems that cause a hoarse voice; diphtheria; epistaxis; inflamed tongue; vomiting blood (from digestive system); hemorrhoids; hemiplegia; pharyngitis; inflammation of the lymph glands; mumps; tonsillitis; otitis; itchy skin problems; thick mucus from the nose; thyroiditis.

KI-6: swelling; allergies; amenorrhea; anosmia; anuria; losing voice; appendicitis; poor blood circulation; ascites; epilepsy; hemorrhoids; blood in the urine; mastitis; melancholia; metritis; seasickness; nephritis; oophoritis; peritonitis; hepatitis; nephrosis; sterility; stomach ulcer.

GB-41: amenorrhea; eczema; anemia; lethargy followed by trembling, eventually leading to emaciation; exhaustion and lethargy; mental retardation; vomiting; deformation of the fingers from rheumatic arthritis or gout; rheumatic pain of the elbows, knees, lumbar or shoulders; menstrual cramps; headache; thrombosis; cataracts; inflammation of the iris; weak eyesight; trigeminal neuralgia; toothache; yawning too much; sprained ankle; inflammation of the bone marrow.

TW-5: joint pain; arteritis; rapid pulse; migraine; inflammation of the skin.

SI-3: spasms of the arms; migraine headache; phobias; loss of ability to speak; torticollis.

BL-62: overexcitement; glaucoma; oversweating; lumbago; sciatica; myopia; torticollis.

Nagatomo and Bachmann Vessel Point Indications

Dr. Nagatomo uses copper on the master points and zinc on the coupled points. Needles are inserted shallowly and perpendicularly. The polarities used depend on the condition, location of the problem and abdominal reactions. Thus, treatments may be unilateral, contralateral or bilateral. There is a twenty minute limit on the treatments.

Chong Mai

Nagatomo: Any diseases that create pain in the abdomen or chest; non-fixed rheumatic symptoms.

Bachmann: Pain that moves; late menses, causing suffering of the heart and increasing heart palpitations leading to insomnia; intestinal spasms.

Yin Wei Mai

Nagatomo: Symptoms similar to those for the chong mai, with a lesser emphasis on pain; heart palpitations; difficulty breathing; phobias.

Bachmann: Symptoms similar to those for the chong mai, with a lesser emphasis on pain; weakness in the heart; palpitations from fear; phobias; easily upset; suddenly talks a lot; easily forgets; easily excited; excessive emotional sympathy (of other people's problems); discomfort or suffering in the chest (*e.g.*, pressure in the chest, stabbing in the heart, palpitations, difficulty breathing, fullness in the chest); borborygmus; no appetite and weight loss with stabbing pain in the intestines at the side of the abdomen or around CV-15 with cold or exhaustion.

Ren Mai

Nagatomo: Emphysema; bronchial catarrh; asthma; diseases of the lower abdomen; skin diseases.

Bachmann: Diseases of the lungs and bronchii (catarrh of upper bronchi, emphysema, bronchitis, pneumonia, nasal polyp, pleurisy, mucositis); diseases of the lower abdomen; diabetes; eczema; tumor.

Yin Qiao Mai

Nagatomo: Peritonitis; hepatitis; nephritis (related to hypoxia or acidosis).

Bachmann: Insomnia; chronic pharyngitis; intestinal poisoning; jaundice; menstrual cramps; uterine bleeding; late labor; white discharge; prostatitis; impotence; bladder spasms; constipation.

Dai Mai

Nagatomo: Pain in any joint; neuralgia; menstrual pain; toothache.

Bachmann: Rheumatic arthritis or neuralgia of the joints, the toes, fingers, shoulders, elbows, wrists, hips, knees, ankles; muscular pain of the neck, head and general muscle pain; menstrual pain or gum pain associated with weakness or tiredness.

Yang Wei Mai

Nagatomo: Mainly any pain on one side of the body (*e.g.* migraine, tendon or tissue pain in the neck); joint inflammation.

Bachmann: Headache; inflammation of the joints; migraine headache; pain in the tendons of the neck; blepharitis; gingivitis; writer's cramp; eye tick; retinitis; poor circulation; low blood pressure; rapid pulse; arteritis; oversensitivity to seasonal change, coldness, etc.; thrombosis; skin inflammation; eczema; pimples; skin swelling; irregular breathing; vomiting blood (from the lungs); bleeding from the nose; stuttering; sprained ankle; bed wetting; heartburn.

Nagatomo comments that symptoms of the yang wei mai are similar to the dai mai, though the symptoms of the yang wei mai are more yang in nature — inflammation, etc.

Du Mai

Nagatomo: Rheumatic arthritis of the spine; inflammation of the joints; neuralgia; head and neck pain; emotional problems.

Bachmann: Rheumatic arthritis of the spine; inflammation of the joints; neuralgia; head and neck pain; emotional problems; overexcitement; nervous breakdown; lack of concentration; insomnia; melancholia; lethargy; epilepsy.

Yang Qiao Mai

Nagatomo: any bleeding problem; stroke; hemiplegia.

Bachmann: any skin bleeding disorder; edema; swelling; cerebrovascular accident; stroke; hemiplegia; tinnitus.

Point Effect Comparisons

In the following sections the point effects described by a variety of sources for the treatment points of each of the extraordinary vessels have been organized by areas, states or symptoms that are most commonly mentioned. Those where no specific ascription to the extraordinary vessels was made are noted by a single point in the "Point" column of the tables. Where the action described was associated with an extraordinary vessel action, this column shows the point pair noted, for example, "PC-6, SP-4." Notations containing a "CC" abbreviation are classical combination treatments where numerous points were used.

The following authors are represented by abbreviations in the "Source" column:

Abbreviation	Source
DC	Zhen Jiu Da Cheng
NB	Nagatomo and Bachmann
JY	Zhen Jiu Ju Ying
NJ	Nanjing CTCM
LS	Li Shi Zhen
SH	Shanghai CTCM
SO	James Tin Yao So

The "miscellaneous" groups are simply lists of the indications for which there were three or fewer matches. Many of these could have been assigned to other groups with interpretation; these were left unascribed to emphasize the main groups. Most matches are reasonably clear. Keep in mind that the intent here is an informal study of the extraordinary vessel treatment points as extraordinary vessel points and as meridian points. Matching itself is not the central issue, just the technique. Indeed, an indication not matching at least one other source is the larger surprise.

Chong Mai Treatment Point Effects

Most of the major categories of chong mai treatments are yin (organ related) in nature or are problems of the front of the body. As we may expect, this group of problems is related to the frontal segments of the body described by Manaka's octahedral view of the extraordinary vessels. Further, most of these problems relate to the pathways of the chong mai or to the combination effects (treatment targets) described by the classical texts. For instance, problems of the abdomen may be seen as a relation to the chong mai pathway. Problems related to alcohol consumption are evocative of the principle that the chong mai meets at "the heart, chest and stomach," the middle warmer, an area generally affected by alcohol consumption. Chest problems are associated with both the chong mai pathway and its meeting at the chest. The eyes and head are on the pathway, the heart is its meeting place.

Of the specific disease states mentioned, the treatment of jaundice may be related to the chong mai affecting the middle warmer, and the amelioration of labor and menstrual problems to its origin in the uterus. Both the spleen and stomach are indicated in nue diseases; the chong mai treatment point is on the spleen meridian and its meeting is at the stomach. The relationship to the stomach is also a potential for curing vomiting. Pain and psychological problems are related to the meeting of the chong mai at the heart, and the function of the heart as the seat of the mind that stores shen.

Category / **Symptoms**	**Points Used**	**Source Text**
abdomen		
abdominal pain	PC-6	SH
abdominal pain	SP-4	NJ
abdomen and sides swollen, full and painful	SP-4, PC-6	JY
abdomen and umbilicus swollen with undigested food	SP-4 (CC)	DC
abdomen discomfort, full, stomach disturbed, nausea and vomiting	SP-4, PC-6	JY
"child pillow pain" (lower abdominal pain)	SP-4, PC-6	JY
dispersed abdominal pain (diarrhea with abdominal pain)	SP-4, PC-6	JY
enlargement of the abdomen	SP-4	SO

one side of abdomen, something hidden in the rib cage	SP-4, PC-6	JY
sudden abdominal pain	SP-4, PC-6	DC
umbilicus and abdomen swollen and painful	SP-4, PC-6	JY

alcohol

alcohol jaundice, body and eyes yellow, deep heart pains	SP-4 (CC)	DC
alcohol or food lumps (yin or yang lumps)	SP-4, PC-6	DC

anus

anal prolapse	SP-4, PC-6	JY
anal prolapse	SP-4	NB
anus is painful following a heavy bout of diarrhea	SP-4, PC-6	JY
rectum prolapsed	PC-6	SH

chest

chest and upper abdomen problems	PC-6	SO
chest pain	PC-6	SH
chronic physical and emotional discomfort in the chest	SP-4, PC-6	DC
diaphragm spasm	PC-6	SH
disease that creates pain in the abdomen or chest	SP-4, PC-6	NB
diseases of the chest	PC-6	SH
fullness and pain inside the chest	SP-4 (CC)	DC
mucus at the diaphragm, chronic physical or emotional discomfort	SP-4 (CC)	DC
mucus heat with a knot inside the chest	SP-4 (CC)	DC
pain at the side of the rib cage	SP-4, PC-6	JY
pressure in the chest	SP-4	NB
problem on one side below the ribs, caused by alcohol	SP-4, PC-6	JY
pulling qi pain in the muscles below the ribs	SP-4, PC-6	JY
shanghan knot in the chest	SP-4, PC-6	JY
sides of the body swollen	SP-4, PC-6	DC
sides of the rib cage swollen and painful	SP-4 (CC)	DC
stabbing pain in the chest	SP-4, PC-6	JY
stagnant qi (choking, rebellious full chest)	SP-4, PC-6	JY
stubborn pain in the sides or below the rib cage	SP-4 (CC)	DC
deep (non-palpable) stabbing pain in the chest	SP-4 (CC)	DC
water, food, qi diseases causing diaphragm problems	SP-4, PC-6	DC

eye

conjunctivitis	SP-4	NB
eyeball inflammation	PC-6	SO
lazy eye	PC-6	NB
night blindness	PC-6	NB
spasming of the eyelid	SP-4	NB

head

head, face swollen	SP-4	SO
feeling of something in the throat	SP-4 (CC)	DC
gingivitis	PC-6	NB
inflammation in the mouth	PC-6	NB
stenosis of the esophagus	PC-6	SO
migraine headache	PC-6	SH
throat swollen and painful	PC-6	SH
tinnitus	SP-4	NB

heart

angina pectoris	PC-6	SH
angina pectoris	PC-6	SO
angina	PC-6	NJ
heat that causes suffering in the heart	SP-4	NB
heart and circulatory problems	SP-4	NB
heart has lost control of the blood	SP-4, PC-6	DC
heart pain; angina	SP-4	NB
heart pain	PC-6	NB
heart palpitations	PC-6	NJ
heart palpitations	SP-4	NB
nine kinds of heart pain and the patient feels cold	SP-4 (CC)	DC
nine kinds of heart pain	SP-4, PC-6	DC
nine kinds of heart pain	SP-4, PC-6	JY
pain below heart, urge to vomit, vomiting after eating	SP-4, PC-6	DC
palpitations	PC-6	SH
rapid palpitations	SP-4	NB
pericarditis and carditis	PC-6	NB
pericarditis	PC-6	SO
pericarditis	SP-4	SO
rheumatic heart diseases	PC-6	SH

intestine

borborygmus	PC-6	NB
borborygmus	SP-4, PC-6	DC
borborygmus	SP-4, PC-6	JY
catarrh of the intestines	PC-6	NB

constipation	SP-4	NB
diarrhea that will not stop, tension and pain in the anus	SP-4 (CC)	DC
diarrhea that will not stop	SP-4, PC-6	JY
diarrhea	SP-4, PC-6	DC
diarrhea	SP-4	NJ
diseases that cause diarrhea	SP-4	NJ
gas	SP-4	SO
hemorrhoid pain	SP-4	NB
hemorrhoids	PC-6	NB
herniated intestines	PC-6	NB
intestinal hemorrhage	SP-4	SO
intestinal spasms	SP-4, PC-6	NB
intestinal spasms	SP-4	NB
intestinal wind with nue and heart pain	SP-4, PC-6	DC
intestines hard, like a drum and abdominal pain	SP-4	SH
stagnant food, food and fluids won't pass, constipation	SP-4, PC-6	JY
wind in the intestines	SP-4, PC-6	JY

jaundice

jaundice	PC-6	SH
jaundice	PC-6	SO
jaundice, four limbs swollen, profuse sweating (clothes wet)	SP-4 (CC)	DC
jaundice, one side of the body more than the other	SP-4 (CC)	DC
grain jaundice, stagnant food causes heart dizziness	SP-4 (CC)	DC
weak jaundice (weakness from too much sex)	SP-4 (CC)	DC

labor

late labor	SP-4	NB
afterbirth, or parts thereof, retained after labor	SP-4, PC-6	DC
bleeding, excess, after labor with dizziness	PC-6	SO
following labor, loss of blood and spontaneous bleeding	SP-4, PC-6	JY
retained placenta	SP-4	SO
retained placenta	PC-6	SO

menses

difficulty with menstruation	SP-4	NB
irregular menses	SP-4 (CC)	DC
irregular menses	SP-4	SH

menses comes late, causing suffering of the heart	SP-4, PC-6	NB

nue

nue and heart pain	SP-4, PC-6	JY
nue of the stomach, always hungry but cannot eat	SP-4 (CC)	DC
nue with first cold then fever	SP-4 (CC)	DC
nue with first fever than cold	SP-4 (CC)	DC
nue with headache, dizziness and vomiting mucus	SP-4 (CC)	DC
nue with heart, chest pain	SP-4 (CC)	DC
nue with high fever that is difficult to eliminate	SP-4 (CC)	DC
nue with soreness of the bones and joints	SP-4 (CC)	DC
nue with thirst (dry mouth included)	SP-4 (CC)	DC
nue of gallbladder, chills, fearfulness, nervous	SP-4 (CC)	DC
nue of heart causing physical, emotional overexcitement	SP-4 (CC)	DC
nue of kidneys (with symptoms like overheating from alcohol)	SP-4 (CC)	DC
nue of liver causing pale blue color, chills, high fever	SP-4 (CC)	DC
nue of lungs causing the heart to be cold, fearful	SP-4 (CC)	DC
nue of spleen causing dread of cold and abdominal pain	SP-4 (CC)	DC

pain

pain associated with surgery	PC-6	SH
pain in the umbilicus	SP-4, PC-6	DC
pain on the yin side of the arm	PC-6	SO
pain that moves	SP-4, PC-6	NB

psychology

hysteria	PC-6	SH
madness	PC-6	NJ
nervous breakdown	PC-6	NB
phobias	PC-6	NB

stomach

catarrh of the stomach or intestines	SP-4	NB
discomfort in middle {warmer}, disturbed stomach, vomiting	SP-4 (CC)	DC
food stagnant in the stomach with stabbing pain	SP-4 (CC)	DC
mucus in the stomach, vomiting clear water	SP-4 (CC)	DC
stomach acutely upset (spasming and/or pain)	SP-4, PC-6	DC
stomach cancer	SP-4	SO

stomach diseases, all kinds	PC-6	SO
stomach spasms	SP-4	NB
stomach spleen disharmony	PC-6	SH
stomach ulcer	SP-4	NB
stomachache	SP-4	SH
stomachache	PC-6	SH
stomachache	SP-4	NJ
stomachache	PC-6	NJ
stomachache	SP-4	SO

vomiting

nausea and vomiting	PC-6	NJ
nausea and vomiting, drooling and dizziness	SP-4 (CC)	DC
vomiting	SP-4	SH
vomiting	PC-6	SH
vomiting	SP-4	NJ
vomiting	SP-4	SO
vomiting and diarrhea	SP-4	SH

miscellaneous

allergies	PC-6	NB
amnesia	PC-6	NB
apoplexy	PC-6	SH
arthritis of the elbow	PC-6	NB
asthma	PC-6	SH
blood pressure problems	PC-6	NB
blood stabbing pain	SP-4, PC-6	JY
children, spleen dispersed (by heat)	SP-4, PC-6	JY
cholera	SP-4	SO
congestion of the brain	PC-6	NB
constantly yawning	SP-4	NB
cystitis	SP-4	NB
decreased appetite	SP-4	SO
difficulty urinating	SP-4	NB
dizziness	PC-6	NB
dropsy	SP-4	SO
endometritis	SP-4	SH
enteritis, chronic and acute	SP-4	SH
epilepsy	PC-6	NJ
epilepsy	SP-4	SO
five kinds of stagnant qi	SP-4 (CC)	DC
food lump (building up) with pain	SP-4, PC-6	JY
foot and ankle pain	SP-4	SH
heart burn	SP-4	NB
gallstone pain	SP-4	NB
hand spasms	PC-6	NB
hepatitis	PC-6	NB
heat diseases	PC-6	NJ

hot diseases	PC-6	NB
hyperthyroidism	PC-6	SH
impotence	PC-6	NB
indigestion	SP-4	NJ
lack of sexual satisfaction during sex	PC-6	NB
liver diseases	SP-4	NB
melancholia and crazed speech	SP-4	SO
melancholia	PC-6	NB
nephritis	PC-6	NB
no appetite	SP-4	NB
non-fixed rheumatic symptoms	SP-4, PC-6	NB
pancreatitis	SP-4	NB
pleurisy	SP-4	SO
rheumatic problems, muscles and joints	SP-4	NB
seizures	SP-4	SH
seizures	PC-6	SH
sharp pain in the back	SP-4	NB
shock	PC-6	SH
spasming pain of the elbows and arms	PC-6	NJ
spleen, overcooling	SP-4	SO
stagnant mucus, drooling and anguished	SP-4, PC-6	JY
stagnant qi, food doesn't move	SP-4, PC-6	JY
stagnant water, alcohol mucus	SP-4, PC-6	JY
stiffness of the penis	SP-4	NB
tidal fevers	SP-4	SH
tidal fevers	PC-6	SH
varicose veins	SP-4	NB
whole body spasms	SP-4	NB
wind pain of the four limbs	SP-4 (CC)	DC
yawning	PC-6	NB
weakness	PC-6	NB

Yin Wei Mai Treatment Point Effects

We can see relationships in the yin wei mai treatment categories that are similar to those for the chong mai. Many are related to organ (yin) problems or problems at the front of the body. Abdominal problems are related to the pathways of both the yin wei mai and chong mai. Chest problems, again, relate to the pathway and the "meeting at the chest." Head problems are also associated with the pathway, heart problems to the meeting at the heart, and psychological problems to the heart function. Stomach problems and vomiting direct our attention to the stomach meeting and hyperthyroidism calls attention to the vessel's pathway through CV-22 and CV-23. Jaundice, alcohol and liver problems relate to the pathway through LV-14 and also the vessel affecting the middle warmer area.

Category / Symptoms	Points Used	Source Text
abdomen		
abdominal pain	PC-6, SP-4	JY
abdominal pain	PC-6	SH
abdominal pain	SP-4	NJ
enlargement of the abdomen	SP-4	SO
congestion of food, lump caused by bleeding, hidden abdominal pain	PC-6 (CC)	DC
no appetite and weight loss with stabbing pain in abdomen	PC-6, SP-4	NB
yin organ lumps, qi lumps, blood lumps on one side of the abdomen	PC-6 (CC)	DC
anus		
anal prolapse	SP-4	NB
anal prolapse in children	PC-6, SP-4	JY
anal prolapse	PC-6, SP-4	DC
anus painful and spasming after much diarrhea	PC-6, SP-4	DC
anus painful following a bout of diarrhea	PC-6, SP-4	JY
difficulty passing stools, straining causing anal prolapse	PC-6 (CC)	DC
five kinds of hemorrhoids, pain is on the outside	PC-6 (CC)	DC
hemorrhoid pain	SP-4	NB
hemorrhoids	PC-6	NB
rectum prolapsed	PC-6	SH
chest		
chest pain	PC-6	SH
chest and upper abdomen problems	PC-6	SO
diaphragm spasm	PC-6	SH
diaphragm, qi and food cannot pass	PC-6, SP-4	JY
difficulty breathing (fullness in the chest)	PC-6, SP-4	NB
discomfort or suffering in the chest, stabbing in the heart	PC-6, SP-4	NB
diseases of the chest	PC-6	SH
during flu, feeling of a knot in the chest	PC-6, SP-4	DC
feeling of fullness in the chest with mucus stagnation	PC-6, SP-4	JY
fullness, stagnation, swelling inside the chest and heart	PC-6, SP-4	DC
knot in the chest	PC-6, SP-4	DC

males, problems below rib cage on one side (alcohol)	PC-6, SP-4	JY
middle warmer full, stagnant, stabbing pains (bilateral)	PC-6, SP-4	DC
pain, lower lateral rib edges, stabbing pain of stomach and heart	PC-6 (CC)	DC
pain in the sides and rib cage	PC-6, SP-4	JY
pressure in the chest	SP-4	NB
shanghan knot in the chest	PC-6, SP-4	JY
stagnant food at the diaphragm	PC-6, SP-4	JY
"two diaphragm," stagnation below the sternum	PC-6, SP-4	JY
(yin) lump at the sides of the body, abdomen	PC-6, SP-4	DC

epilepsy

epilepsy	PC-6	NJ
epilepsy	SP-4	SO
five kinds of epilepsy, bubbly saliva in the mouth	PC-6 (CC)	DC

head

congestion of the brain	PC-6	NB
conjunctivitis	SP-4	NB
constantly yawning	SP-4	NB
difficulty swallowing	PC-6, SP-4	DC
eyeball inflammation	PC-6	SO
gingivitis	PC-6	NB
head, face swollen	SP-4	SO
inflammation in the mouth	PC-6	NB
lazy eye	PC-6	NB
migraine headache	PC-6	SH
night blindness	PC-6	NB
spasming of the eyelid	SP-4	NB
stenosis of the esophagus	PC-6	SO
throat swollen and painful	PC-6	SH
tinnitus	SP-4	NB

heart

angina pectoris	PC-6	SH
angina pectoris	PC-6	SO
angina	PC-6	NJ
heart and chest, stagnation and fullness	PC-6, SP-4	JY
heart and circulatory problems	SP-4	NB
heart and gallbladder empty, attacked by shock	PC-6 (CC)	DC
heart and rib cage swollen and painful	PC-6, SP-4	JY

heart empty and gallbladder cold, whole body shaking	PC-6 (CC)	DC
heart pain; angina	SP-4	NB
heart pain	PC-6	NB
heart palpitations	PC-6, SP-4	NB
heart palpitations	SP-4	NB
heart palpitations	PC-6	NJ
heart qi empty or lost, laughing or singing	PC-6 (CC)	DC
heat that causes suffering in the heart	SP-4	NB
palpitations from fear	PC-6, SP-4	NB
palpitations	PC-6, SP-4	NB
palpitations	PC-6	SH
pericarditis and carditis	PC-6	NB
pericarditis	SP-4	SO
pericarditis	PC-6	SO
rapid palpitations	SP-4	NB
rheumatic heart diseases	PC-6	SH
weakness in the heart	PC-6, SP-4	NB
women, a lump (side) that is painful, with heart pain	PC-6, SP-4	DC

intestines

borborygmus	PC-6, SP-4	NB
borborygmus	PC-6, SP-4	DC
borborygmus	PC-6, SP-4	JY
borborygmus	PC-6	NB
catarrh of the intestines	PC-6	NB
constipation	SP-4	NB
diarrhea and "slippery intestines"	PC-6, SP-4	JY
diarrhea	PC-6, SP-4	DC
diarrhea	SP-4	NJ
diseases that cause diarrhea	SP-4	NJ
gas	SP-4	SO
herniated intestines	PC-6	NB
intestinal hemorrhage	SP-4	SO
intestinal spasms	SP-4	NB
intestine wind and bleeding from the anus	PC-6, SP-4	JY
intestines hard, like a drum and abdominal pain	SP-4	SH
large intestine empty and cold, anal prolapse	PC-6 (CC)	DC

labor

bleeding, excess, after labor with dizziness	PC-6	SO
retained placenta	SP-4	SO
retained placenta	PC-6	SO
late labor	SP-4	NB

psychology

amnesia	PC-6	NB
easily excited	PC-6, SP-4	NB
easily forgets	PC-6, SP-4	NB
easily upset	PC-6, SP-4	NB
emptiness in the heart, paranoia; shen & thinking anxious	PC-6 (CC)	DC
"heart surprised," babbling, speech unclear	PC-6 (CC)	DC
"heart surprised," leading to collapse and coma	PC-6 (CC)	DC
"heart type" of idiot, unending sadness and crying	PC-6 (CC)	DC
forgetfulness, mental unclarity (like senility)	PC-6 (CC)	DC
hysteria	PC-6	SH
madness, "heart surprised"	PC-6 (CC)	DC
madness	PC-6	NJ
nervous breakdown	PC-6	NB
overly emotionally sympathetic (to other people's problems)	PC-6, SP-4	NB
phobias	PC-6, SP-4	NB
phobias	PC-6	NB
suddenly talks a lot	PC-6, SP-4	NB

stomach

catarrh of the stomach or intestines	SP-4	NB
fullness and discomfort inside, stomach cold evil	PC-6 (CC)	DC
stomach cancer	SP-4	SO
stomach diseases, all kinds	PC-6	SO
stomach spasms	SP-4	NB
stomach spleen disharmony	PC-6	SH
stomach ulcer	SP-4	NB
stomachache	SP-4	SH
stomachache	PC-6	SH
stomachache	SP-4	NJ
stomachache	PC-6	NJ
stomachache	SP-4	SO
spleen and stomach empty, cold, vomiting and nausea	PC-6 (CC)	DC
spleen and stomach qi empty, heart and abdomen swollen	PC-6 (CC)	DC
spleen, overcooling	SP-4	SO

vomiting

irregular vomiting	PC-6, SP-4	JY
nausea and vomiting	PC-6	NJ
vomiting and diarrhea	SP-4	SH
vomiting	SP-4	SH

vomiting	PC-6	SH
vomiting	SP-4	NJ
vomiting	SP-4	SO

miscellaneous

alcohol mucus, "stagnant pain"	PC-6, SP-4	JY
allergies	PC-6	NB
apoplexy	PC-6	SH
arthritis of the elbow	PC-6	NB
asthma	PC-6	SH
blood pressure problems	PC-6	NB
blood stabbing pain in women	PC-6, SP-4	JY
breathing	PC-6, SP-4	NB
cholera	SP-4	SO
congealed, stagnant qi, easily loses control	PC-6 (CC)	DC
cystitis	SP-4	NB
damage from alcohol	PC-6, SP-4	DC
decreased appetite	SP-4	SO
difficulty urinating	SP-4	NB
difficulty with menstruation	SP-4	NB
dizziness	PC-6	NB
dropsy	SP-4	SO
endometritis	SP-4	SH
enteritis, chronic and acute	SP-4	SH
foot and ankle pain	SP-4	SH
gallstone pain	SP-4	NB
hand spasms	PC-6	NB
heart burn	SP-4	NB
heat diseases	PC-6	NJ
hepatitis	PC-6	NB
hot diseases	PC-6	NB
hyperthyroidism	PC-6	SH
impotence	PC-6	NB
inability to transform rice and grains	PC-6, SP-4	JY
indigestion	SP-4	NJ
irregular menstruation	SP-4	SH
jaundice	PC-6	SH
jaundice	PC-6	SO
liver diseases	SP-4	NB
lump in the inguinal crease	PC-6, SP-4	JY
lump pain	PC-6, SP-4	JY
melancholia and crazed speech	SP-4	SO
melancholia	PC-6	NB
nephritis	PC-6	NB
no appetite	SP-4	NB
nue disease	PC-6, SP-4	DC
organ poisoning, swollen pain, blood in the stools	PC-6 (CC)	DC
pain associated with surgery	PC-6	SH

pain on the yin side of the arm	PC-6	SO
pancreatitis	SP-4	NB
pleurisy	SP-4	SO
lack of sexual satisfaction during sex	PC-6	NB
rheumatic problems, muscles and joints	SP-4	NB
seizures	SP-4	SH
seizures	PC-6	SH
shanghan injury by cold invasion	PC-6, SP-4	JY
sharp pain in the back	SP-4	NB
shock	PC-6	SH
spasming pain of the elbows and arms	PC-6	NJ
stagnant food will not disperse, slow wasting of the body	PC-6 (CC)	DC
stagnation, lump, deep heart or anguished pain	PC-6 (CC)	DC
stiffness of the penis	SP-4	NB
tidal fevers	SP-4	SH
tidal fevers	PC-6	SH
varicose veins	SP-4	NB
weakness	PC-6	NB
whole body spasms	SP-4	NB
yawning	PC-6	NB
yin and yang organs empty and cold, both sides of the body painful	PC-6 (CC)	DC

Ren Mai Treatment Point Effects

Like the chong and yin wei mai, the general focus of the ren mai is frontal and internal, as is predicted by octahedral theory. We may also see many ren mai categories that relate to the ren mai pathway—point combination targets, LU-7 (lung meridian relationships) and KI-6 (kidney meridian relationships). Abdominal problems may be seen as treated through the ren mai pathway; blood problems, especially menstrual blood problems, to the trajectory of its pathway and its origin in the uterus. Similarly, labor or menstrual problems may result from imbalances of the ren mai vessel. Chest problems implicate the pathway and the "meeting at the supporter of the lungs, at the throat and diaphragm." Problems of the head, nose, genitals, peritoneum or anus also relate to the pathway, and problems of the throat, such as cough, relate to both the vessel trajectory and its meeting at the throat. There are also relationships to the KI-6 point and the kidney meridian itself. Invasion problems, wind or skin problems could be related to the LU-7—lung meridian functions.

Category / Symptoms	Points Used	Source Text
abdomen		
abdomen cold & painful inside, diarrhea that will not stop	LU-7 (CC)	DC
lower abdomen pain	KI-6	SO
pinching pain in abdomen & umbilicus	LU-7, KI-6	JY
stagnation in lower abdomen, related to head	LU-7	NB
stagnation on one side of abdomen caused by alcohol, food cannot pass	LU-7, KI-6	JY
stagnation on one side of abdomen with pain	LU-7, KI-6	JY
swollen and painful abdomen, diarrhea that will not stop	LU-7 (CC)	DC
umbilical and abdominal pain	LU-7 (CC)	DC
arms		
arms, shoulders, chest or back cold	LU-7	SO
arms and legs contracting, spasming in children attacked by wind	LU-7 (CC)	DC
hand or arm pain	LU-7	NJ
wrist joint diseases	LU-7	SH
blood		
blood circulation poor	KI-6	NB
blood in the urine	KI-6	NB
blood lump in women	LU-7, KI-6	JY
blood lump, pain or emotional distress post partum	LU-7, KI-6	JY
blood lump, post partum with pain or emotional distress	LU-7 (CC)	DC
blood problems and cold umbilicus	LU-7, KI-6	DC
reckless bleeding and dizziness caused by blood problems	LU-7 (CC)	DC
chest		
abscess of the breast	LU-7, KI-6	DC
abscessed breast, swollen and painful, baby vomiting	LU-7 (CC)	DC
asthma	LU-7	SH
chest pain	LU-7	NJ
chest, coughing, panting, cold mucus, tight, contracting pain	LU-7 (CC)	DC

chest, front between the nipples, is red, swollen, painful	LU-7 (CC)	DC
chest, loud raspy breathing, diaphragm tight and painful	LU-7 (CC)	DC
chest, lower portion uncomfortable	LU-7	SO
chest, panting, shortness of breath, mucus, qi stagnant	LU-7 (CC)	DC
chest, stagnant knot between chest and diaphragm	LU-7 (CC)	DC
chest, stagnant pain inside, unable to swallow	LU-7 (CC)	DC
chest, swelling, pain or abscess on the sides	LU-7, KI-6	JY
dyspnea	LU-7	SO
loud panting, qi full, lungs feel swollen, cannot lie down	LU-7 (CC)	DC
phlegm in the chest	LU-7	SO
mastitis	KI-6	NB
small pimple on the nipple (probably purulent)	LU-7 (CC)	DC
panting	LU-7	SH
panting	LU-7	NJ
women, respiratory or lower abdominal stagnation	LU-7	NB

children

convulsions in children	LU-7	SO
children, eyes open, fixed, arms and legs spasming, bubbling saliva	LU-7 (CC)	DC

cough

chronic cough, blood and mucus in the saliva	LU-7 (CC)	DC
cough	LU-7	NJ
coughing	LU-7	SH
coughing	LU-7	SO
coughing with cold mucus	LU-7, KI-6	JY
hematuria and cough with mucus	LU-7, KI-6	DC

digestion

bloody faeces	LU-7, KI-6	JY
borborygmus and diarrhea	LU-7, KI-6	JY
cannot digest (rice and grains)	LU-7, KI-6	JY
cold pain and diarrhea	LU-7, KI-6	JY
constipation	KI-6	NJ
constipation	LU-7, KI-6	JY
stagnant food and digestive problems	LU-7, KI-6	JY
white or red diarrhea, inside of abdomen cold, pain	LU-7 (CC)	DC

head

abscess or pimple in the mouth, halitosis	LU-7 (CC)	DC
chronic runny nose	LU-7 (CC)	DC
ear, sound like insects in (tinnitus)	LU-7 (CC)	DC
eye pain	KI-6	SH
face, paralysis	LU-7	SO
five kinds of lumps in the neck	LU-7 (CC)	DC
headache	LU-7	SH
inflamed tongue	LU-7	NB
nasal polyps or other growths in the nose	LU-7 (CC)	DC
neck stiff	LU-7	SH
mouth awry	LU-7	SH
mouth cannot open	LU-7	SO
mucosa, diseases of	LU-7	NB
mumps	LU-7	NB
nose runny (watery), skin feels rough, sneezing	LU-7 (CC)	DC
nose stuffed, cannot discern smells	LU-7 (CC)	DC
nose, runny, dirty turbid mucus	LU-7 (CC)	DC
nose, thick mucus	LU-7	NB
pharyngitis	KI-6	SH
pharyngitis	LU-7	NB
pharynx	LU-7	SH
paralysis, face	LU-7	SH
sputum, drops of blood in	LU-7, KI-6	DC
teeth swollen and painful	LU-7, KI-6	JY
terrible halitosis	LU-7 (CC)	DC
throat blocked	KI-6	SH
throat dry	KI-6	SH
throat dry	KI-6	SO
throat numb	LU-7	SO
throat sore	LU-7	NJ
throat swollen and painful	LU-7, KI-6	JY
thyroiditis	LU-7	NB
tonsillitis	LU-7	NB
tonsillitis	KI-6	SH
tonsillitis	KI-6	SO
toothache	LU-7, KI-6	DC
voice, losing of	KI-6	NB
voice, problems that cause hoarseness	LU-7	NB

heart

heart (inside) feels anxious or uncomfortable	LU-7 (CC)	DC
heart and abdomen pain	LU-7, KI-6	JY
heart pain with warm diarrhea	LU-7, KI-6	JY
heart	LU-7, KI-6	DC

hemiplegia

hemiplegia	LU-7	SO
hemiplegia	LU-7	SH
hemiplegia	KI-6	SH
hemiplegia	LU-7	NB

hemorrhoids

hemorrhoids	KI-6	NB
hemorrhoids	LU-7	NB
hemorrhoids	LU-7, KI-6	DC
hemorrhoids, itchy, painful bleeding	LU-7, KI-6	JY

labor

agalactia	LU-7	NB
fetus dies, will not deliver	LU-7, KI-6	JY
labor difficult	KI-6	SH
labor, inability to speak after	LU-7, KI-6	JY
labor, lumbar pain following	LU-7, KI-6	JY
labor, madness after	LU-7, KI-6	JY
miscarriage with retention of part of the afterbirth	LU-7, KI-6	DC
placenta, retained	KI-6	SO

limbs

ankle joint pain	KI-6	SO
elbow or wrist weak	LU-7	SO
foot swollen	KI-6	SO
four limbs lazy, tired	KI-6	SO
four limbs, sudden swelling (Marie's disease)	LU-7	SO
lymph glands swollen in the inguinal joint	LU-7, KI-6	JY
legs swollen	KI-6	NJ
limbs, acute edema of	LU-7	SH

menstruation

amenorrhea	KI-6	NB
menses irregular	KI-6	NJ
menstrual problems, unusual menses, discharge	LU-7	NB
menstruation irregular	KI-6	SH
menstruation irregular	KI-6	SO
spotting between menses, irregular bleeding, unable to lactate	LU-7 (CC)	DC

stomach

extreme heat in stomach, delirium, vomiting	LU-7 (CC)	DC
stomach, intestine pain	LU-7, KI-6	JY
ulcer	KI-6	NB

sha

black sha, abdominal pain, headache, fever, chills	LU-7 (CC)	DC
black and white sha, headache, thirst, large intestine diarrhea	LU-7 (CC)	DC
white sha, abdominal pain, vomiting or diarrhea, limbs cold	LU-7 (CC)	DC

urination

urination frequent	KI-6	NJ
urination, burning sensation	LU-7	SO
urine, blood and semen in	LU-7	SO
urine, blood in	LU-7, KI-6	DC
urine, blood in	LU-7, KI-6	JY
urine, blood in	LU-7	SH
urine, difficulty passing	KI-6	NJ
urine, inability to pass	LU-7, KI-6	JY

vagina

vaginal discharge	KI-6	SH
vaginal itching	KI-6	SO
vaginal spasm	KI-6	SO

vomiting

vomiting blood (from digestive system)	LU-7	NB
vomiting saliva with pus and blood	LU-7, KI-6	JY
vomiting, bubbly saliva	LU-7	SO
vomiting, ceaseless	LU-7, KI-6	JY

wind

attack by wind, red face, high fever headache	LU-7 (CC)	DC
attack by wind, susceptible to cold, coughing and panting	LU-7 (CC)	DC

external wind injures the four limbs, fever, headache	LU-7 (CC)	DC
rash, wind	LU-7	SH

miscellaneous

absolute heat in triple warmer, mouth abscess or pimple	LU-7 (CC)	DC
acne	LU-7	NB
allergies	KI-6	NB
anosmia	KI-6	NB
anuria	KI-6	NB
anus is swollen	LU-7, KI-6	DC
appendicitis	KI-6	NB
ascites	KI-6	NB
attacked by cold with fever	LU-7 (CC)	DC
beri-beri	KI-6	NJ
delirium	LU-7	SO
diphtheria	LU-7	NB
edema	KI-6	SH
epilepsy	KI-6	NB
epilepsy	KI-6	NJ
epistaxis	LU-7	NB
genital itching	KI-6	SH
genitals itchy	KI-6	NJ
hepatitis	KI-6	NB
hernia, acute	KI-6	SO
hot disease (that hasn't been cured)	LU-7, KI-6	JY
insomnia	KI-6	NJ
insomnia	KI-6	SH
internal heat and anuria	LU-7 (CC)	DC
laughing	LU-7	SO
lipomas	LU-7	NB
lumbago	LU-7, KI-6	DC
lumbar pain	LU-7, KI-6	DC
lump (any)	LU-7, KI-6	JY
lymph gland inflammation	LU-7	NB
malaria, chronic	KI-6	SO
melancholia	KI-6	NB
metritis	KI-6	NB
nephritis	KI-6	NB
nephrosis	KI-6	NB
neurasthenia	KI-6	SH
nue	LU-7, KI-6	DC
oophoritis	KI-6	NB
otitis	LU-7	NB
penis pain	LU-7	SO
peritonitis	KI-6	NB
psychosis	KI-6	SH
red or white discharge	KI-6	NJ

scrofula	LU-7	SO
seasickness	KI-6	NB
seizures	KI-6	SH
skin itchy	LU-7	NB
skin problems that cause peeling	LU-7	NB
small intestine "qi pinching" pain	LU-7, KI-6	JY
sterility	KI-6	NB
swelling	KI-6	NB
tuberculosis	LU-7	SO
urticaria	LU-7	SH
uterus prolapsed	KI-6	SH
vanished kidneys	LU-7 (CC)	DC
vanished middle	LU-7 (CC)	DC
vanished spleen	LU-7 (CC)	DC

Yin Qiao Mai Treatment Point Effects

The yin qiao mai treatment focus also justifies its place in octahedral theory, frontal and internal. Yin qiao mai categories relate to the pathway, point combination targets, and LU-7, KI-6, lung and kidney meridians. Abdominal problems can be seen in association with the yin qiao mai pathway, alcohol problems to its "meeting at the diaphragm." The diaphragm lies in the middle warmer region, the area most affected by alcohol problems. Chest and coughing symptoms are related to the pathway and its "meeting at the supporter of the lungs, throat and diaphragm." Obstetric, gynecologic, genital and urinary problems figure in the ren mai pathway and the ren mai to yin qiao mai connection. Problems of the head, epilepsy and hemiplegia may also relate to imbalances in the vessel itself. Intestinal problems and worms may be treated with the lung—large intestine correlation accessed through the LU-7—luo point relationship. Similarly, skin problems may be treated through the lung meridian; water, edema and kidney problems through the kidney relationships.

Category / Symptoms	Points Used	Source Text
abdomen		
abdomen & umbilicus, pinching pain	LU-7, KI-6	JY
abdomen, feeling of fullness and discomfort	KI-6, LU-7	JY

cold pain of the lower abdomen, voluminous urination	KI-6 (CC)	DC
heart and abdomen swollen and big	KI-6 (CC)	DC
stagnation in lower abdomen, related to head	LU-7	NB
pain in lower abdomen	KI-6, GB-34	LS
pain in lower abdomen	KI-6	SO
umbilicus and abdomen pain	KI-6, LU-7	JY

alcohol

alcohol lump in abdomen and umbilicus	KI-6, LU-7	DC
alcoholism in males, lump on one side, food stagnation	KI-6, LU-7	JY
bi symptoms caused by alcohol	KI-6, LU-7	JY
lump, yin type, caused by alcohol	KI-6, LU-7	JY

arms

arms, shoulders, chest or back cold	LU-7	SO
elbow or wrist weak	LU-7	SO
hand or arm pain	LU-7	NJ
wrist joint diseases	LU-7	SH

beri-beri

beri-beri	KI-6	NJ
deficient kidney beri-beri, red and swollen, high fever	KI-6 (CC)	DC
dry beri-beri, patella, internal ankle, fingers, or toes painful	KI-6 (CC)	DC

bladder

bladder qi pain	KI-6, LU-7	DC
bladder qi stagnant with pain	KI-6, LU-7	JY
strong, acute pain of the bladder (seven kinds)	KI-6 (CC)	DC

blood

blood circulation poor	KI-6	NB
blood dizziness in women	KI-6, LU-7	JY
blood in the urine	KI-6	NB
blood lump in women	KI-6, LU-7	JY

chest

chest pain, feeling of qi pushing or pressing	KI-6 (CC)	DC
chest pain	LU-7	NJ

chest, lower portion uncomfortable	LU-7	SO
dyspnea	LU-7	SO

childbirth

pillow pain, stagnant blood after labor	KI-6, LU-7	JY
difficult labor, baby disturbs the mother's mind	KI-6 (CC)	DC
difficult labor	KI-6 (CC)	DC
difficult labor	KI-6, LU-7	DC
difficult labor	KI-6	SH
agalactia	LU-7	NB
lactation problem, acute pain in lower abdomen or back, heart	KI-6 (CC)	DC
pain in the abdomen and umbilicus after labor, constant discharge	KI-6 (CC)	DC
retained placenta	KI-6	SO
retained afterbirth	KI-6, LU-7	JY

cough

coughing	LU-7	SH
coughing	LU-7	SO
cough	LU-7	NJ

epilepsy

epilepsy	KI-6, GB-34	LS
epilepsy	KI-6	NB
epilepsy	KI-6	NJ

head

eye pain	KI-6	SH
esophagus and trachea feel stagnant like something stuck	KI-6 (CC)	DC
inflamed tongue	LU-7	NB
facial paralysis	LU-7	SO
facial paralysis	LU-7	SH
headache	LU-7	SH
mouth awry	LU-7	SH
mouth cannot open	LU-7	SO
mucosa, diseases of	LU-7	NB
neck stiff	LU-7	SH
nose, thick mucus	LU-7	NB
numbness of the skin	KI-6, GB-34	LS
pharyngitis	KI-6	SH
pharyngitis	LU-7	NB
pharynx swollen	LU-7	SH

plum pit qi in the throat	KI-6, LU-7	DC
swollen lymph glands in the inguinal joint	KI-6, LU-7	JY
throat sore	LU-7	NJ
throat blocked	KI-6	SH
throat dry	KI-6	SH
throat dry	KI-6	SO
throat numb	LU-7	SO
throat swollen, feels closed	KI-6, LU-7	JY
throat, feeling of something stuck in	KI-6, LU-7	DC
thyroiditis	LU-7	NB
tonsillitis	LU-7	NB
tonsillitis	KI-6	SH
tonsillitis	KI-6	SO

hemiplegia

hemiplegia	KI-6	SH
hemiplegia	LU-7	SH
hemiplegia	LU-7	NB
hemiplegia	LU-7	SO

intestine

borborygmus, diarrhea, abdominal pain	KI-6, LU-7	JY
borborygmus	KI-6, LU-7	DC
constipation	KI-6	NJ
constipation	KI-6, LU-7	JY
hemorrhoids	KI-6	NB
hemorrhoids	LU-7	NB
intestine, bleeding from the wall of	KI-6, LU-7	JY
small intestine swollen and full	KI-6, LU-7	JY
undigested food (in the stools)	KI-6, LU-7	JY
painful stomach, hard stools	KI-6, LU-7	DC
wind in the intestines (bloody stools), bleeding from the anus	KI-6, LU-7	DC

limbs

acute edema of limbs	LU-7	SH
ankle joint pain	KI-6	SO
four limbs, face and eyes swollen	KI-6 (CC)	DC
four limbs lazy, tired	KI-6	SO
feet hot	KI-6, LU-7	JY
foot swollen	KI-6	SO
limbs, legs swollen	KI-6	NJ
sudden swelling of four limbs (Marie's disease)	LU-7	SO
weak energy in old people, arms and legs hard to move	KI-6 (CC)	DC

menses

amenorrhea	KI-6	NB
menses irregular	KI-6	NJ
menstrual problems, unusual menses, discharge	LU-7	NB
menstruation irregular	KI-6	SH
menstruation irregular	KI-6	SO

skin

skin itchy	LU-7	NB
skin problems that cause peeling	LU-7	NB
rash, wind	LU-7	SH

urination

anuria	KI-6	NB
blood and semen in urine	LU-7	SO
blood in urine	LU-7	SH
difficulty passing urine	KI-6	NJ
incontinence of urine, blood in urine, sexual organ pain	KI-6 (CC)	DC
incontinence or feeling of stagnation, urine drips, does not stream	KI-6 (CC)	DC
urinary incontinence	KI-6, LU-7	DC
urination frequent	KI-6	NJ
urination with burning sensation	LU-7	SO
urination, cold pain	KI-6, LU-7	JY
urination rough, dripping, won't pass	KI-6, LU-7	JY
urticaria	LU-7	SH

uterus

uterus prolapsed	KI-6	SH
monthly water imbalance, pain in umbilicus or abdomen	KI-6 (CC)	DC
chronic coldness of the uterus	KI-6 (CC)	DC

vagina

vaginal discharge	KI-6	SH
vaginal itching	KI-6	SO
vaginal spasm	KI-6	SO

vomiting

vomiting and diarrhea	KI-6, LU-7	DC

vomiting blood (from digestive system)	LU-7	NB
vomiting with bubbly saliva	LU-7	SO
yellow food (in the vomit)	KI-6, LU-7	DC
food and fluids immediately vomited, upside down stomach	KI-6, LU-7	JY
nausea and vomiting	KI-6, LU-7	JY

worms

blood worms	CV-4 (CC)	DC
both qi and blood worms	KI-6 (CC)	DC
qi worms	SP-4	DC
stone worms	ST-44	DC
water worms	KI-6 (CC)	DC

women

blood and qi weak	KI-6 (CC)	DC
constipation in women	KI-6 (CC)	DC
continuous discharge in women	KI-6, GB-34	LS
headache, dizziness, pain in kidney and lower abdomen in women	KI-6 (CC)	DC
respiratory system or lower abdomen stagnation, women	LU-7	NB
spleen qi problems, worms in women	KI-6 (CC)	DC
weakness in women, skinny body, red & white discharge	KI-6 (CC)	DC

miscellaneous

acne	LU-7	NB
allergies	KI-6	NB
anosmia	KI-6	NB
appendicitis	KI-6	NB
ascites	KI-6	NB
asthma	LU-7	SH
cold, damp beri-beri, fever with a lot of pain	KI-6 (CC)	DC
coma and lumps	KI-6, LU-7	DC
convulsions in children	LU-7	SO
deficient spleen with food lump, stagnant food, etc.	KI-6, LU-7	JY
deficient symptoms of "ocean tide"	KI-6, LU-7	JY
deficient yang, the patient is like a corpse	KI-6 (CC)	DC
delirium, vomiting or diarrhea, arms and legs cramping	KI-6 (CC)	DC
delirium	LU-7	SO
diphtheria	LU-7	NB

dreams of sex with a (Chinese) demon, spermatorrhea	KI-6 (CC)	DC
epistaxis	LU-7	NB
genital itching	KI-6	SH
genitals itchy	KI-6	NJ
edema	KI-6	SH
heat in the five hearts	KI-6 (CC)	DC
hepatitis	KI-6	NB
hernia, acute	KI-6	SO
hot or cold symptoms	KI-6, GB-34	LS
imbalance of water, kidney swelling on one side	KI-6 (CC)	DC
insomnia	KI-6	NJ
insomnia	KI-6	SH
laughing	LU-7	SO
lipomas	LU-7	NB
lymph gland inflammation	LU-7	NB
malaria, chronic	KI-6	SO
mastitis	KI-6	NB
melancholia	KI-6	NB
metritis	KI-6	NB
mumps	LU-7	NB
nephritis	KI-6	NB
nephrosis	KI-6	NB
neurasthenia	KI-6	SH
oophoritis	KI-6	NB
otitis	LU-7	NB
panting	LU-7	SH
panting	LU-7	NJ
penis pain	LU-7	SO
peritonitis	KI-6	NB
phlegm in the chest	LU-7	SO
pressure in the heart, stressed (suffers shock)	KI-6 (CC)	DC
psychosis	KI-6	SH
pulling pain from lumbar, iliac crest to sexual organs	KI-6, GB-34	LS
qi lump	KI-6, LU-7	JY
red or white discharge	KI-6	NJ
scrofula	LU-7	SO
seasickness	KI-6	NB
seizures	KI-6	SH
separated blood, simple abdomen, qi panting	KI-6 (CC)	DC
simple abdomen, worm swelling, qi panting	KI-6 (CC)	DC
spermatorrhea, white unclear sperm, frequent urination	KI-6 (CC)	DC
stagnant qi	KI-6, LU-7	JY
sterility	KI-6	NB

stomach ulcer	KI-6	NB
swelling	KI-6	NB
tuberculosis	LU-7	SO
vision, "stars in vision"	KI-6	SO
voice, losing of	KI-6	NB
voice, problems that cause hoarseness	LU-7	NB
whole body swollen, full and puffy (water)	KI-6 (CC)	DC

Dai Mai Treatment Point Effects

The dai mai treatment targets are much more structural and musculoskeletal, and more strongly directed toward the upper body than the front or internal parts. Thus dai mai would relate to the yang areas of the octahedron. Many dai mai treatment categories are related to the pathway of the dai mai or yang wei mai, but the areas most often affected relate to the dai mai. Arm problems can be seen to relate to the yang wei mai pathway, as can problems of the feet. Foot problems may as well relate to the gallbladder meridian. Problems of the hands can be seen in relation to the triple warmer pathway. Problems of the head and legs may indicate both yang wei mai pathway and the areas most affected by the dai mai—yang wei mai combination, or where they meet. The areas most affected with lumbar problems are on the dai mai pathway. Menstrual problems can be seen to relate to the dai mai pathway through BL-23. Problems of the ears and eyes remind us of the "meeting at the lateral aspects of the eyes and behind the ears." Surface invasion, or skin problems are within the scope of the principle that the yang extraordinary vessels "mainly treat diseases. . . that are superficial."

Category / **Symptoms**	**Points Used**	**Source Text**
arm		
arm and elbow cramp	TW-5	SO
arm, elbow, difficulty bending, stretching	TW-5	NJ
arm and leg tightness, spasming	GB-41, TW-5	JY
arm cold bi pain	GB-41 (CC)	DC
arm pain, shoulder and back problems	GB-41 (CC)	DC
arms and legs numb	GB-41 (CC)	DC
arms and legs spasming	GB-41 (CC)	DC

body

body itching	GB-41 (CC)	DC
body numbness	GB-41, TW-5	JY
body swollen	GB-41, TW-5	JY
body weak, no energy in the four limbs	GB-41 (CC)	DC
four limbs, gout	GB-41 (CC)	DC
four limbs, lack of control	GB-41, TW-5	JY
four limbs, moving pain (joints or meridians)	GB-41 (CC)	DC
pain, fever, numbness and spasms	GB-41, TW-5	DC
paralysis	TW-5	SH

chest

breast abscessed	GB-41	SH
breast carbuncle	GB-41	SO
carbuncles behind clavicle and armpit	GB-41	SO
cheek and chin pain	GB-41, TW-5	JY
chest feels full	GB-41	SO
chest pain with chills	GB-41	SO
rib cage painful	GB-41	NJ
rib cage painful	TW-5	NJ
rib area swollen	GB-41	SO
rib pain	TW-5	SH
rib pain	GB-41	SH
side and rib pain	GB-41, TW-5	JY
stabbing pain below rib cage with palpable lump	GB-41 (CC)	DC
mastitis	GB-41	SH

ears

deafness	GB-41, TW-5	DC
deafness	GB-41, TW-5	JY
deafness	TW-5	SH
deafness	TW-5	SO
deafness	TW-5	NJ
tinnitus	TW-5	SH
tinnitus	TW-5	NJ

eyes

cataracts	GB-41	NB
conjunctivitis	GB-41	SH
eyes dizzy	GB-41	SO
eyes red and swollen with vertigo	GB-41, TW-5	DC
eyes red, cold tearing	GB-41, TW-5	JY
eyes red, swollen, painful	TW-5	NJ

eyes swollen and painful	GB-41, TW-5	JY
eye pain, lateral canthus	GB-41	NJ
eyesight weak	GB-41	NB
iris inflammation	GB-41	NB

feet

ankles red and swollen (external)	GB-41 (CC)	DC
ankle sprained	GB-41	NB
chronic swelling, pain on dorsum of foot	GB-41 (CC)	DC
foot swelling, damp	GB-41	SH
heat in soles of feet	GB-41 (CC)	DC
heat on dorsum of feet, pain in joints	GB-41 (CC)	DC
swelling and pain of dorsum of feet	GB-41	NJ
swelling, pain on top of foot	GB-41, TW-5	JY
toes spasming, tight, unable to open	GB-41 (CC)	DC
toes spasming with pain	GB-41	NJ

hands

finger pain, hand weak	TW-5	SO
finger pain, inhibits grasp	TW-5	SH
fingers numb, pain bending and straightening	GB-41 (CC)	DC
fingers deformed from rheumatic arthritis or gout	GB-41	NB
hands, fingers, pain	TW-5	NJ
hand tremors	TW-5	SH
hands and arms, bone pain	GB-41 (CC)	DC
hands and feet hot	GB-41, TW-5	JY
hands and feet numb	GB-41, TW-5	JY
hands and fingers numb	GB-41, TW-5	JY
hands shaking, unable to hold anything	GB-41 (CC)	DC
hands, heat with pain fingers	GB-41 (CC)	DC

head

back of neck, chin swelling	GB-41, TW-5	DC
base of skull sore	GB-41	SO
Bell's palsy	GB-41, TW-5	JY
head and back of neck red, swelling, painful	GB-41 (CC)	DC
head and eye dizziness	GB-41, TW-5	JY
head itchiness, swelling, severe dandruff	GB-41, TW-5	JY
head wind (thunder)	GB-41, TW-5	JY
head wind pain	GB-41, TW-5	DC
head wind	GB-41, TW-5	JY
head, top swollen	GB-41, TW-5	JY

headache (migraine)	TW-5	SH
headache	GB-41	SH
headache	GB-41	NB
headache	TW-5	NJ
migraine	TW-5	NB
neck stiff	TW-5	SH
throat swollen and painful	GB-41, TW-5	JY
throat swollen	GB-41, TW-5	DC
throat swollen	TW-5	SH
trigeminal neuralgia	GB-41	NB
toothache	GB-41, TW-5	DC
toothache	GB-41, TW-5	JY
toothache	GB-41	NB

hemiplegia

hemiplegia of the hands and legs, cannot raise	GB-41, TW-5	DC
hemiplegia	TW-5	SH

joints

inguinal joint pain	GB-41, TW-5	JY
joints painful, upper limbs	TW-5	SH
joints, all painful	GB-41 (CC)	DC
joint pain	TW-5	NB
elbows, knees, lumbar or shoulders, pain	GB-41	NB

legs

knees and shins painful	GB-41 (CC)	DC
knees red, swollen, sore	GB-41 (CC)	DC
leg and knee swollen	GB-41, TW-5	JY
leg painful (different areas at different times)	GB-41	SO
legs shaking, difficulty walking	GB-41 (CC)	DC

lumbar

lumbar and groin pain	GB-41 (CC)	DC
lumbar pain from strain	GB-41 (CC)	DC
lumbar pain, deficiency, dampness, stagnant	GB-41 (CC)	DC
kidney lumbar pain, difficult, strained movements	GB-41 (CC)	DC

thigh

thigh and bladder pain	GB-41 (CC)	DC

thigh pain, sides swollen, imbalance (one side)	GB-41, TW-5	DC
thigh, cold bi pain	GB-41 (CC)	DC

menses

menstruation	GB-41	SH
amenorrhea	GB-41	NB
menstruation irregular	GB-41	SO
menses irregular	GB-41	NJ
menstrual cramps	GB-41	NB

miscellaneous

anemia	GB-41	NB
arteritis	TW-5	NB
bone marrow inflammation	GB-41	NB
constipation	TW-5	SH
cold (common)	TW-5	SH
dyspnea and difficulty walking	GB-41	SO
excessive secretion (female) during intercourse	GB-41	SO
enuresis	TW-5	SH
eczema	GB-41	NB
fever (high)	TW-5	SH
gout pains	GB-41 (CC)	DC
heat diseases	TW-5	NJ
floating wind (itching and muscular tension)	GB-41, TW-5	DC
itchiness and floating wind	GB-41, TW-5	JY
lethargy, trembling, leading to emaciation	GB-41	NB
malaria	GB-41	SO
mental retardation	GB-41	NB
muscle spasms and bone pain	GB-41, TW-5	JY
shanghan	GB-41, TW-5	JY
skin inflammation	TW-5	NB
scrofula	GB-41	SH
thrombosis	GB-41	NB
overtired and lethargic	GB-41	NB
pneumonia	TW-5	SH
parotitis	TW-5	SH
pulse rapid	TW-5	NB
tibia sore	GB-41	SO
stroke (attack by wind), cannot raise the arms and legs	GB-41, TW-5	JY
vertigo	GB-41	SH
urine dripping	GB-41	NJ
vomiting	GB-41	NB
yawning too much	GB-41	NB

Yang Wei Mai Treatment Point Effects

As with the dai mai, most of the symptoms and signs relate to structural or upper body problems, the yang areas. Many of the main categories concern the yang wei pathway (arm and foot problems); the triple warmer meridian pathway (hand problems); the areas the yang wei mai "meets at" or "mainly treats" (eye, ear, head and back problems).

Category / Symptoms	Points Used	Source Text
arm		
arm and elbow cramp	TW-5	SO
arms and legs numb, painful, weak	TW-5, GB-41	JY
arms cold, painful	TW-5, GB-41	JY
arms red, swollen from shoulders down, joints sore	TW-5 (CC)	DC
body		
body swollen after labor	TW-5, GB-41	JY
four limbs unable to move smoothly	TW-5, GB-41	JY
four limbs, joints, swelling, pain	TW-5, GB-41	JY
inability to raise the four limbs with head wind	TW-5, GB-41	DC
joints painful, upper limbs	TW-5	SH
joints swollen, painful, knees cold	TW-5, GB-41	DC
muscle, tendon or bone pain	TW-5, GB-41	JY
night sweating	TW-5, GB-41	JY
spasms and numbness following apoplexy	TW-5 (CC)	DC
paralysis	TW-5	SH
wind after labor	TW-5, GB-41	JY
back		
back and groin, bone, muscle problems	TW-5, GB-41	DC
lumbar and back swelling, pain	TW-5, GB-41	JY
lumbar and hip joint pain	TW-5, GB-41	JY
blood		
epistaxis	TW-5, GB-41	JY
epistaxis that does not stop, reckless bleeding	TW-5 (CC)	DC

reckless blood, congested heat of six yang organs	TW-5 (CC)	DC
vomiting blood, weakness, no energy, rebellious qi	TW-5 (CC)	DC
vomiting blood, congested heat of five yin organs	TW-5 (CC)	DC
vomiting blood, dizziness, unconsciousness, almost comatose	TW-5, CC	DC
vomiting blood, epistaxis, hot, reckless blood	TW-5 (CC)	DC
vomiting blood, yin overcomes the yang	TW-5 (CC)	DC

chest

breast abscessed	GB-41	SH
breast carbuncle	GB-41	SO
carbuncles behind clavicle and armpit	GB-41	SO
chest feels full	GB-41	SO
chest pain with chills	GB-41	SO
rib area swollen	GB-41	SO
rib pain	GB-41	SH
rib pain	TW-5	SH
lymph glands swollen (chest to armpit)	TW-5 (CC)	DC
mastitis	GB-41	SH

ears

deafness	TW-5	SH
deafness	TW-5	SO
deafness, qi stagnation and pain in the ear	TW-5 (CC)	DC
ear ringing, itchy or sore	TW-5 (CC)	DC
earlobe (left side) swollen, knot or lump	TW-5 (CC)	DC
earlobe (right side) swollen, knot or lump	TW-5 (CC)	DC
earlobe red swollen and painful	TW-5 (CC)	DC
tinnitus	TW-5	SH

eyes

conjunctivitis	GB-41	SH
eyes dizzy	GB-41	SO
eyes red, swollen, infected	TW-5, GB-41	DC
eyes red, swollen, pimples at outer canthus (in wind)	TW-5 (CC)	DC
eyes swollen	TW-5, GB-41	JY
eyes swollen, itchy, tearing (in wind)	TW-5 (CC)	DC
eyes red, painful, hot	TW-5 (CC)	DC

eyes, infection of the surface unable to open	TW-5 (CC)	DC
eyes, pain	TW-5, GB-41	JY
sore, red eyes	TW-5, GB-41	JY
shadow on the eyes (cataract)	TW-5, GB-41	JY
tearing in a wind	TW-5, GB-41	JY

hands

finger pain, hand weak	TW-5	SO
hand and arm pain	TW-5, GB-41	JY
hand tremors	TW-5	SH
hands and feet hot, numb, night sweats	TW-5, GB-41	DC
hands and feet hot	TW-5, GB-41	JY
finger joint pain, cannot bend	TW-5, GB-41	JY
finger joints painful, unable to bend or stretch	TW-5 (CC)	DC
finger pain, inhibits grasp	TW-5	SH

head

head, back of neck pain	TW-5, GB-41	JY
head, back of neck, around eyes, pain	TW-5, GB-41	DC
head, pain on the top	TW-5 (CC)	DC
headache	GB-41	SH
headache (migraine)	TW-5	SH
headache, heavy head, unable to lift the head	TW-5 (CC)	DC
headwind	TW-5, GB-41	JY
headwind with shaking and pain	TW-5, GB-41	JY
mouth, sore or abscess	TW-5 (CC)	DC
neck stiff	TW-5	SH
neck, large lump	TW-5 (CC)	DC
neck, red and swelling	TW-5 (CC)	DC
throat swollen	TW-5	SH
thunder headwind	TW-5, GB-41	JY
thunder headwind, dizziness, drooling	TW-5 (CC)	DC
tongue contracted, difficulty speaking	TW-5 (CC)	DC
tongue swollen, puffy heavy, high fever, unable to speak	TW-5 (CC)	DC
tongue tight, stiff, difficulty speaking, white buds	TW-5 (CC)	DC
toothache, both sides swollen and painful	TW-5 (CC)	DC

lips split, bleeding, dry, sore	TW-5 (CC)	DC
pain in lower canine teeth, cheeks, neck red, swollen	TW-5 (CC)	DC
pain in upper canine teeth, unable to open mouth	TW-5 (CC)	DC
skull, base sore	GB-41	SO

feet

foot, swelling, damp	GB-41	SH
ankle, internal bone red, swelling, painful	TW-5 (CC)	DC
leg painful (different areas at different times)	GB-41	SO
toe joint pain, unable to walk	TW-5 (CC)	DC

miscellaneous

cold knees	TW-5, GB-41	DC
common cold	TW-5	SH
constipation	TW-5	SH
dyspnea and difficulty walking	GB-41	SO
enuresis	TW-5	SH
excessive secretion (female) during intercourse	GB-41	SO
fever (high)	TW-5	SH
flu with spontaneous sweating	TW-5, GB-41	DC
hemiplegia	TW-5	SH
malaria	GB-41	SO
menstruation irregular	GB-41	SH
menstruation irregular	GB-41	SO
parotitis	TW-5	SH
pneumonia	TW-5	SH
scrofula	GB-41	SH
shanghan, with spontaneous sweating	TW-5, GB-41	JY
shanghan, with superficial fever	TW-5, GB-41	JY
tetanus	TW-5, GB-41	JY
tibia sore	GB-41	SO
vertigo	GB-41	SH
vertigo, "mucus rebellious head dizziness,"	TW-5 (CC)	DC
vomiting will not stop	TW-5 (CC)	DC

Du Mai Treatment Point Effects

The main categories of du mai treatments center, like the dai and yang wei mai, on the more structural and upper body problems – again, more yang sections of Dr. Manaka's octahedron. The internal pathway of the du mai through the brain accounts for its effects on problems of the back, head and possibly psychological problems and dizziness as well. It "meets at" the nose next to the eyes, the ears, the arms and the small intestine and bladder meridians. Thus, it is able to affect problems of the eyes, ears, arms, hands and legs. SI-3 and BL-62 lie on the small intestine and bladder meridian pathways, which may further account for the effects on the arms, hands and legs. It "mainly" affects problems of the thighs and problems that are superficial, such as sweating dysfunction.

Category / Symptoms	Points Used	Source Text
arm		
arm and elbow cramps	SI-3	SO
arm spasms	SI-3	NB
arm upper pain	SI-3	NJ
arms and legs numb	SI-3, BL-62	DC
arms and legs numb	SI-3, BL-62	JY
arms and legs shaking	SI-3, BL-62	JY
arms and legs tense, spasms	SI-3, BL-62	JY
arms and legs tight, spasming, difficulty stretching	SI-3 (CC)	DC
arms and legs weak, unable to walk	SI-3 (CC)	DC
arms and legs, spasms, contractions or shaking	SI-3, BL-62	DC
shin, knee and thigh pain	SI-3, BL-62	JY
wrist pain	SI-3	NJ
back		
back and thigh pain	BL-62	NJ
back pain (low)	SI-3	SH
lumbago	BL-62	NB
lumbar and back pain and tension	SI-3, BL-62	JY
pain, lower back and legs	BL-62	SH

ears

deaf-mutism	SI-3	SH
deafness, hardness of hearing	SI-3 (CC)	DC
deafness	SI-3	SH
deafness	SI-3	SO
tinnitus	BL-62	SH
tinnitus	SI-3	SH

dizziness

dizziness	BL-62	SH
dizziness	BL-62	NJ
dizziness	BL-62	SO

epilepsy

epilepsy	SI-3	SO
epilepsy	BL-62	SO
epilepsy, vomiting bubbly saliva	SI-3, BL-62	JY
epilepsy	BL-62	NJ
epilepsy	SI-3, BL-62	DC

eyes

eyes red and painful	SI-3	SH
eyes red and swollen, tearing in wind	SI-3 (CC)	DC
eyes tear in wind	SI-3, BL-62	JY
eyes, swollen, red	SI-3, BL-62	JY
glaucoma	BL-62	NB
conjunctivitis (with film over eyes)	SI-3	SO
membrane on the eye	SI-3	SH
myopia	BL-62	NB
eyebrows, pain at both ends	SI-3 (CC)	DC

hands

finger spasms	SI-3	NJ
finger spasm	SI-3	SH
hands numbness and spasming	SI-3, BL-62	JY

head

head and eyes dizzy	SI-3 (CC)	DC
cheek and chin swelling and pain	SI-3, BL-62	JY

cheek, jaw, glands red and swelling	SI-3 (CC)	DC
head and eyes droop	SI-3 (CC)	DC
head and neck tight, pulled backwards	SI-3 (CC)	DC
head, neck tense, hard, tight	SI-3 (CC)	DC
headache (migraine)	SI-3	NB
headache, dizziness from alcohol	SI-3 (CC)	DC
headache, eyes swollen, tearing	SI-3, BL-62	DC
headache, lateral and midline	BL-62	SH
headache	BL-62	SH
headache	BL-62	NJ
headache	SI-3	NJ
headache	BL-62	SO
headwind pain	SI-3, BL-62	JY
headwind, unilateral or bilateral	SI-3 (CC)	DC
neck pain	SI-3	NJ
neck stiff	SI-3	SO
neck stiff	SI-3	SH
neck tension	SI-3, BL-62	DC
neck, tension, pain, immobility	SI-3 (CC)	DC
teeth (gums) and throat swollen	SI-3, BL-62	DC
throat spasms	SI-3, BL-62	JY
throat stagnant	SI-3, BL-62	JY
throat, feeling of something stuck	SI-3 (CC)	DC
tonsillitis (both tonsils)	SI-3 (CC)	DC
tonsillitis (one tonsil)	SI-3 (CC)	DC
toothache	SI-3, BL-62	JY
toothache	SI-3 (CC)	DC
mouth and eyes awry	BL-62	SH

jaundice

jaundice	SI-3	SH
jaundice	SI-3	NJ
jaundice	SI-3	SO

leg

knee or thigh pain, radiates to lumbar or back	SI-3, BL-62	DC
knees and shin, swelling, pain	SI-3, BL-62	JY
leg pain (lower)	BL-62	SO
arthritis of the ankles	BL-62	SH

psychology

insanity	BL-62	SH
madness	BL-62	NJ
madness	BL-62	SO

madness	SI-3	SO
phobias	SI-3	NB
psychosis	BL-62	SH
psychosis	SI-3	SH
overexcitement	BL-62	NB

sweating

excessive sweating	SI-3	SO
inability to sweat	SI-3, BL-62	JY
night sweating	SI-3, BL-62	DC
night sweats	SI-3	SH
nights sweats	SI-3	SO
oversweating	BL-62	NB
profuse night sweating	SI-3, BL-62	JY

miscellaneous

ability to speak declining	SI-3	NB
after labor, spontaneous sweating, dread of wind	SI-3, BL-62	JY
arteriosclerosis	BL-62	SO
attacked by wind (stroke), unable to speak	SI-3, BL-62	JY
epistaxis	SI-3	SO
external wind (epilepsy), inability to speak	SI-3, BL-62	DC
external wind	SI-3, BL-62	DC
coughing, panting, cold mucus	SI-3 (CC)	DC
heat diseases with no sweat	SI-3	NJ
hemiplegia	BL-62	SH
difficulty standing up	BL-62	SO
influenza	SI-3, BL-62	DC
malaria (with cold and high fever)		
malaria	SI-3	SH
Meniere's disease	BL-62	SH
meningitis	BL-62	SH
muscles, tendons, bones pain	SI-3, BL-62	JY
palpitations	BL-62	SH
scabies	SI-3	SO
sciatica	BL-62	NB
seizures	BL-62	SH
septicemia, tetanus, high fever, tension	SI-3 (CC)	DC
shanghan headache	SI-3, BL-62	JY
shanghan, pain, stiffness back of neck	SI-3, BL-62	JY
shanghan	SI-3, BL-62	JY

shoulder pain	SI-3	NJ
stroke, loss of speech	BL-62	SH
tetanus	SI-3, BL-62	DC
tetanus	SI-3, BL-62	JY
tetanus	SI-3 (CC)	DC
tidal fever	SI-3	SH
torticollis	BL-62	NB
torticollis	SI-3	NB
uterus pain	BL-62	SO

Yang Qiao Mai Treatment Point Effects

The main focus of the yang qiao mai is musculoskeletal, structural and upper body, as we would expect. The pathway of the yang qiao mai would account for treatment of the head, arms and back; its internal pathway through the brain for stroke, dizziness and psychological problems. It "meets" at the lateral edges of the bridge of the nose, next to the eyes, the back of the neck and at the ears. Thus problems of the nose, such as epistaxis, of the ears, such as deafness, and of the eyes and neck may all be treated. It "mainly" affects problems that are superficial, which could explain its effects on surface infections and invasions.

Category / **Symptoms**	**Points Used**	**Source Text**
apoplexy		
ability to speak declining	SI-3	NB
ability to speak declining	BL-62 (CC)	DC
loss of speech	BL-62	SH
unable to concentrate	BL-62 (CC)	DC
apoplexy	GB-39	LS
eyes rolled up into the head	BL-62 (CC)	DC
four limbs spasming	BL-62 (CC)	DC
hemiplegia	BL-62 (CC)	DC
arm		
arm & elbow cramps	SI-3	SO
arm spasms	SI-3	NB
arms & hands pain	BL-62, SI-3	JY
arms & legs can not raise	BL-62, SI-3	JY
arms & legs numb	BL-62, SI-3	DC

arms & legs numb	BL-62, SI-3	JY
arms & legs spasm	BL-62, SI-3	JY
cold arms	BL-62, SI-3	JY
upper arm pain	SI-3	NJ
upper arms cold	BL-62, SI-3	DC

back

back & thigh pain	BL-62	NJ
pain (low)	SI-3	SH
lumbago	BL-62	NB
lumbar and back stiff and painful	BL-62, SI-3	JY
lumbar and back tight when bending	BL-62, SI-3	DC
lumbar area lesion	BL-62 (CC)	DC
lumbar or back pain	GB-39	LS
lumbar pain, hard to move leg	BL-62 (CC)	DC
lumbar pain, neck and back pain	BL-62 (CC)	DC
lumbar pain	BL-62 (CC)	DC
pain lower back and legs	BL-62	SH
sciatica	BL-62	NB

deafness

deafness	BL-62, SI-3	DC
deafness	BL-62, SI-3	JY
deafness	SI-3	SH
deafness	SI-3	SO
deafness with mutism	SI-3	SH

dizziness

dizziness	BL-62	SH
dizziness	BL-62	NJ
dizziness	BL-62	SO

epilepsy

epilepsy	BL-62	SO
epilepsy	SI-3	SO
epilepsy	BL-62, SI-3	DC
epilepsy	BL-62, SI-3	JY
epilepsy	BL-62	NJ
epilepsy	GB-39	LS

epistaxis

epistaxis	BL-62, SI-3	DC
epistaxis	BL-62, SI-3	JY
epistaxis	SI-3	SO

eyes

conjunctivitis, with film over eyes	SI-3	SO
eyes red and painful	BL-62, SI-3	DC
eyes red and painful	SI-3	SH
eyes red and swollen	BL-62, SI-3	JY
eyebrow bone pain	BL-62, SI-3	JY
glaucoma	BL-62	NB
membrane on eyes	SI-3	SH
myopia	BL-62	NB

head

head & face - spontaneous sweating	BL-62, SI-3	JY
head hard to bend down or over	BL-62 (CC)	DC
head wind	BL-62, SI-3	JY
headache	BL-62, SI-3	DC
headache	BL-62	SH
headache	BL-62	NJ
headache	SI-3	NJ
headache	BL-62	SO
headache - lateral and midline	BL-62	SH
headache - migraine	SI-3	NB
itching pain - headwind	BL-62, SI-3	JY
sweating of head	BL-62, SI-3	DC
thunder head wind	BL-62, SI-3	DC

hemiplegia

facial hemiplegia	BL-62 (CC)	DC
hemiplegia	BL-62 (CC)	DC
hemiplegia	BL-62	SH
hemiplegia	GB-39	LS
hemiplegia following apoplexy	BL-62 (CC)	DC

jaundice

jaundice	SI-3	SH
jaundice	SI-3	NJ
jaundice	SI-3	SO

limb

joint pain	BL-62 (CC)	DC
joint pain	BL-62, SI-3	DC
joint pain	BL-62, SI-3	JY
joint swelling and pain	BL-62, SI-3	JY
arthritis of the ankles	BL-62	SH
neck or nape hard to move	BL-62 (CC)	DC

neck pain	SI-3	NJ
neck stiff	SI-3	SO
shoulder pain	SI-3	NJ
stiff neck	SI-3	SH
thighs and knees swelling and pain	BL-62, SI-3	JY
thighs swollen and tight	BL-62, SI-3	DC
leg pain (lower)	BL-62	SO
wrist pain	SI-3	NJ

psychology

madness	BL-62	NJ
madness	BL-62	SO
madness	SI-3	SO
insanity	BL-62	SH
phobias	SI-3	NB
psychosis	BL-62	SH
psychosis	SI-3	SH
overexcitement	BL-62	NB

malaria

malaria (with cold and high fever)		
malaria	SI-3	SH
tidal fever	SI-3	SH

balance

body numb or tight	GB-39	LS
body swollen	BL-62, SI-3	JY
body tension	BL-62 (CC)	DC
difficulty standing up	BL-62	SO
hand and leg weak	BL-62 (CC)	DC
mouth and eyes awry	BL-62	SH
mouth tight, unable to open	BL-62 (CC)	DC
one side of the body full, swollen	BL-62, SI-3	DC
one side of the body painful	BL-62 (CC)	DC
one side of the body weak	BL-62 (CC)	DC

sweat

excessive sweating	SI-3	SO
oversweating	BL-62	NB
spontaneous sweating after labor	BL-62, SI-3	JY
spontaneous sweating	BL-62, SI-3	DC
night sweats	SI-3	SH
night sweats	SI-3	SO

spasms

face spasming (one side)	BL-62 (CC)	DC
four limbs spasming after stroke	BL-62 (CC)	DC
arm spasms	SI-3	NB
finger spasms	SI-3	NJ
finger spasm	SI-3	SH
seizures	BL-62	SH

infection

abscess lumbar area	BL-62 (CC)	DC
abscess	BL-62 (CC)	DC
abscess breast (superficial large)	BL-62, SI-3	DC
poisoning of the back of the hand and arm	BL-62 (CC)	DC
poisoning on the dorsum of the foot	BL-62 (CC)	DC
poisoning on the dorsum of the hand	BL-62 (CC)	DC
poisoning on the face	BL-62 (CC)	DC
tetanus	BL-62, SI-3	JY

invasion

dread of cold	GB-39	LS
dread of wind after labor	BL-62, SI-3	JY
dread of wind	BL-62, SI-3	DC
heat diseases with no sweat	SI-3	NJ
shanghan, injury by cold with spontaneous sweating	BL-62, SI-3	JY
shanghan, injury by cold	BL-62, SI-3	JY

miscellaneous

arteriosclerosis	BL-62	SO
breast pain - pain when breast feeding	BL-62, SI-3	JY
crying	GB-39	LS
tinnitus	BL-62	SH
tinnitus	SI-3	SH
torticollis	BL-62	NB
torticollis	SI-3	NB
meningitis	BL-62	SH
Meniere's disease	BL-62	SH
palpitations	BL-62	SH
scabies	SI-3	SO
uterus pain	BL-62	SO

Conclusions

Let us return to the questions at the beginning of the chapter, that we may now propose some answers:

> *1. Is an extraordinary vessel action involved only when both the master and coupled point pair is stimulated?*
>
> *2. Is the stimulation of the extraordinary vessel points by some specific type of stimulation the key that determines if an extraordinary vessel action will be induced?*
>
> *3. Do the body's energies respond to the stimulation of an extraordinary vessel point through the extraordinary vessels only when there is a related imbalance?*

The first question can be addressed at two levels: the perspective of point effects and the perspective of meridian—extraordinary vessel relationships.

On reviewing the literature it is apparent that some of the effects of the eight treatment points described in earlier books referred to the extraordinary vessels and thus to treatment of both the master and coupled points. In later texts these were described as single point effects. The structure of the *Zhen Jiu Da Cheng* treatments imply that the extraordinary vessel effects may be obtained by stimulation of only one extraordinary vessel point in conjunction with other body points. Though it would be tenuous at best to generalize that this assumption would always be correct, the therapeutic reputation of the points has been continuous. The books and practitioners that do not mention the extraordinary vessel relationships nonetheless used the single points with clinical success.

We suggest that stimulation of the extraordinary vessel points will effect results and that this effect may be seen to relate to points as "meridian points" as well as extraordinary vessel points. The structural and topological basis of the extraordinary vessels as demonstrated by Dr. Manaka is based on this theory. Stimulation of SI-3 and BL-62 to activate the du mai—yang qiao mai pair for the treatment of back disorders cannot be divorced from the effects of these two points on the bladder and small intestine meridians and thus the back. It is more than coincidence that these two points were selected as du mai—yang qiao mai treatment points. The attempt to separate structure and function is practically senseless. How is it possible to separate the energetics of the body from the structure of the body? The central position of the extraordinary vessels, their intimate connection to the energetic center of the body, and their function as the "oceans and seas" of the branch meridians argues against such a separation.

Without attempting a broad generalization, we can direct discussion of the second of our rhetorical questions to the clinical evidence that the type of stimulation given to the eight points does vary the effects produced. Needling the the eight points with stainless steel needles produces a different effect than when we needle with copper or zinc needles. When we apply aluminum—south and gold—north magnets, we again produce different results. The specific results may be different; yet regardless of the stimulation, we may generalize that these results are obtained at a deep energetic level. The similarity or difference of the terms by which we label the effects should not distract us from the importance of the extraordinary vessels as a means of access to profound functions.

The third question is particularly interesting and particularly difficult to address, for its resolution involves some of the issues raised by the first and second questions. If the extraordinary vessels affect and reflect both deep energetic and structural imbalances, then we must consider the relationship between structure and function. The ren and du mai are the oceans of yin and yang, the chong mai the ocean of blood, the twelve meridians, the five yin and six yang organs. Somehow the eight extraordinary vessels encompass the meridian—organ system and yet function, at least in part, separately. Without diagnosing a ren mai imbalance or intending to affect the ren mai, can we treat LU-7, with the intention of treating the luo point of the lung meridian, and *not* produce some action that is related to the ren mai? Probably not. Even this terse answer raises another question. If we clearly diagnose a lung or lung luo meridian problem, how do we determine that this problem is outside the sphere of influence of the ren mai? Again, the answer is terse; we cannot.

The trouble begins with the problem statement. The "actions and effects" of points are, like channels, syndromes and disease names, organizing concepts, not fixed bioenergetic realities. They form the conceptual map by which we orient our therapeutic searches. A point is a "meridian point" or an "extraordinary vessel point" only in our discussions. Within the interacting biosphere of the human body an acupoint is a complex entity the stimulation of which may increase or decrease the flow of energy in a certain subset of the organism's energetic metabolism, or transmit information that modifies the reactions of other subsystems and functions.

Body structure, itself a complex result of the energies and signals that govern growth, muscular tonus, skeletal alignment and the relative, balanced stresses of the body's fascial sheaths and ligaments, may be altered by changes in both the metabolic and informational energy systems. The reverse is as true, that the body's structure may alter the strength and distribution of bioelectrical and hormonal "messages" and metabolic abilities. It is therefore reasonable to presume that the effects of any point's stimulation will depend on both the point stimulation and the condition of the systems stimulated. Both sender and receiver are essential. It is in these considerations that the power of the model provided by Dr. Manaka's theories is most apparent. The topological and octahedral models of the extraordinary vessels give us a most complete and clinically useful overview that avoids the unjustified separation of structure and energy, vessel and meridian.

Notes

[1] *Zhen Jiu Xue*, the Nan Jing Medical school textbook, 1979. References for each point are as follows: LU-7, p. 22; SP-4, p. 45; SI-3, p. 55; BL-62, p. 71; KI-6, p. 78; PC-6, p. 86; TW-5, p. 89; GB-41, p. 103.

[2] *Secondary Vessels of Acupuncture*. England: Thorsons Publishing, 1983.

[3] Nagatomo's symptomologies come from Tsugio Nagatomo, *Nagatomo M.P. Shinkyu Kuowa Hachijuhachi Syu*, p. 31. Bachmann's symptomologies come from p. 32 of the same.

Appendix One
Electromagnetic Therapeutics

Mr. Ito's style of treatment using the pointer machine for electromagnetic therapy is highly extensible. The following sections provide supplemental information that is useful when combining this treatment style with five element diagnosis and treatment, scar therapy and zone therapy. You can see from the principles, techniques and styles described that there are many ways of using the extraordinary vessels and the pointer machine. While the variety may be somewhat overwhelming at first, if your are thorough and systematic in your diagnosis, it is possible to obtain extremely good results.

Five Element Diagnosis

Five element diagnosis requires a variety of information to ensure accuracy. While knowledge of the entire system is necessary, this section lists techniques that are used by experienced practitioners to increase the efficiency of their treatments. This review of five element diagnosis is offered with the intention of directing the attention of the practitioner toward techniques that will increase their efficacy and contribute to the development of combination treatments based on the extraordinary vessels. As such, these suggestions are particularly useful when combining five element diagnosis with extraordinary vessel diagnosis and classical five element treatments with electromagnetic therapy. The most common situations are those most necessary to develop and sophisticate.[1]

Pulse Diagnosis

Most Oriental five element practitioners use the pulse diagnosis system that comes from Chapter 18 of the *Nan Jing*. The relative strengths of the pulses in each of the six positions and the relative depth of the pulse in each position are the main diagnostic signs.[2]

This system diagnoses the condition of each of the twelve meridians. The yang meridians reflect in the superficial pulse and the yin meridians reflect in the deeper pulse. According to the *Nan Jing*, these correspondences are:

		Inch	Bar	Foot
Left	Superficial	Small Intestine	Gall Bladder	Bladder
	Deep	Heart	Liver	Kidney
Right	Superficial	Large Intestine	Stomach	(fire of) Triple Warmer
	Deep	Lung	Spleen	Master of Heart Pericardium

While there is a complete system of diagnosis based on the individual pulse qualities found at each of these positions, we do not recommend that beginners place much emphasis on their attempts to discern these qualities. This is difficult for beginners and can take years to master. It is more effective, and enhances learning, to focus on the depth at which the pulse may be felt and to concentrate on how wide or narrow, weak or strong a pulse is found to be.

In general, *Nan Jing* five element diagnosis concentrates on deficiency rather than excess. This is partly because of the *Nan Jing* dictum to tonify before dispersing and partly from the general predominance of deficiency in the patient population. The principle of building qi is a practical first step. Some practitioners report that most of their patients are either spleen, liver or kidney deficient, and that these three conditions are by far the more common deficiencies. Thus, a concentration on the width and depth of the pulse will not only reliably reveal the most usual information, but will also serve as a foundation for experience that will lead to skill in the more subtle aspects of pulse discernment.

Good, accurate diagnosis of the pulse is also helpful in determining the efficacy of treatment during and after its ministration. If the treatment is working as you planned, the pulses will balance, or at least, ameliorate. Regularly rechecking the pulse is an essential step in most combination treatments.

Abdominal diagnosis

Abdominal palpation is the most important component of making a diagnosis by the five elements. Not only is it capable of indications as subtle as those determined by the pulse, and therefore able to confirm pulse diagnosis, it is able to supply information that leads to greater skill at pulse diagnosis itself. Confirmation is essential for inexperienced practitioners and routinely sought by the experienced. Further, the signs found on the abdomen often change rapidly and thus provide another accurate means of gauging treatment progress. Because there is a considerable base of abdominal palpation information, much of it from modern authors who have provided clear explanations in modern languages,[3] testing the abdomen allows the practitioner access to a variety of successful methods and clinical rules.

It is most important to palpate the entire abdomen. Palpate in the numbered sequence shown in the following illustration, down the center line and the lines on the left side of the abdomen. Then, palpate upward on the lines of the right side of the abdomen, across each subcostal region, sweeping along to the edge of the iliac and pelvic bones. In all places remember to begin with shallower pressure and repeat with deeper pressure.[4]

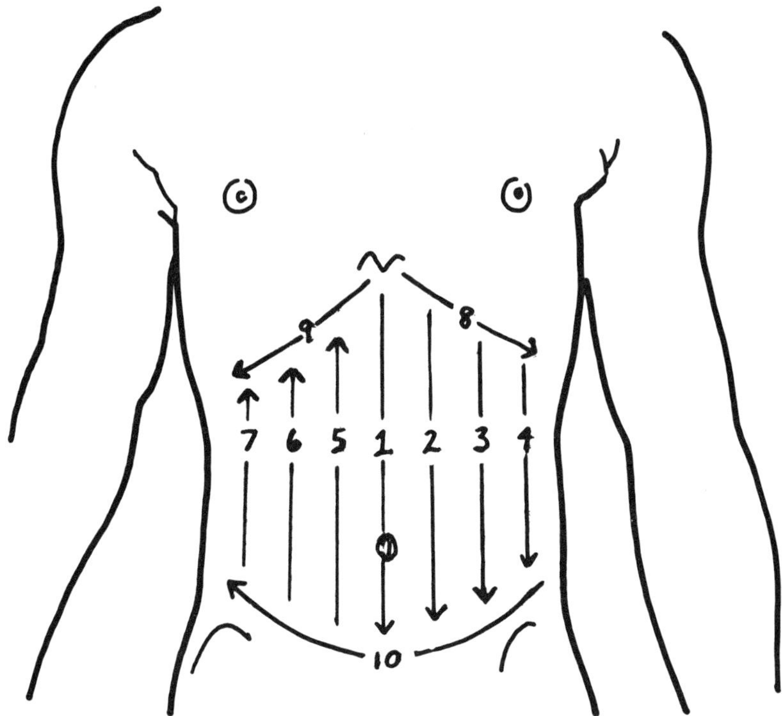

Figure 40

It is important to note that abdominal reactions may be more important and useful than pulse signs, that pulses may be affected by many unrelated phenomena, where changes in the abdomen may be more specific to the treatment. As the classics warn us, pulse diagnosis requires specific conditions. Abdominal reactions, usually points of tension, pain, flaccidity or some physiological indication, tend to be more robust and objective.

The following notes describe a variety of signs derived from the experience of different practitioners. For each element deficiency there are notations of the following signs:

- Abdominal reactions,
- Body point reactions,
- Toe nail, finger nail, foot and toe shapes,
- Other observable signs,
- Symptom complexes.

Diagnostic Notes

Diagnosis is performed in a manner similar to the diagnosis of extraordinary vessel imbalance by constructing a diagnostic pattern. Usually the abdomen and pulse play the more important role in the diagnosis; accompanying signs and symptoms are used to confirm the diagnosis. This emphasis is not always applicable, but as a "rule of thumb" it is sufficient. Try to diagnose the meridian—element that is deficient, or most deficient. When treating using the pointer machine magnetic therapies, it is best to focus on the single, most important deficiency. There are patients for whom it is difficult to distinguish between two element—meridian deficiences. In these cases both may be treated, though the use of magnetic therapy may not be the method of choice. Classical five element treatments should be considered. If a single, clear element deficiency cannot be ascertained, it may be better to use yet another set of principles for diagnosis and treatment.

Spleen Deficiency

Palpation

Pulsing from CV-7 to CV-9;
Pressure pain or tightness around the navel, especially around CV-7;
A chopstick-shaped tightness from CV-7 to CV-12;
Puffiness around the navel;
Pressure pain or tension below the ribs on the left side;
Pressure pain, looseness or weakness around SP-3, SP-4.

Keep in mind that pulsing at CV-9 can also indicate kidney deficiency; it may be necessary to differentiate.

Accompanying Signs

Toes of an unhealthy color;
Tension or tightness between the shoulder blades;
The eyes swell easily or feel swollen;
The fingertips are dry and crack easily;
Fatigue or easily tired;
Legs swell after walking;
Frequent flatulence;
Tense or swollen lower abdomen;
A desire to lay down frequently;
Frequent yawning;
Sleeps lightly, easily awakened;
Alternating constipation and diarrhea;
Sores and cracks on the lips, particularly the corners of the mouth;
Canker sores behind the lips;
Dry lips;
Weakness similar to hypoglycemia;
Sleepiness after eating.

Signs on the Feet:

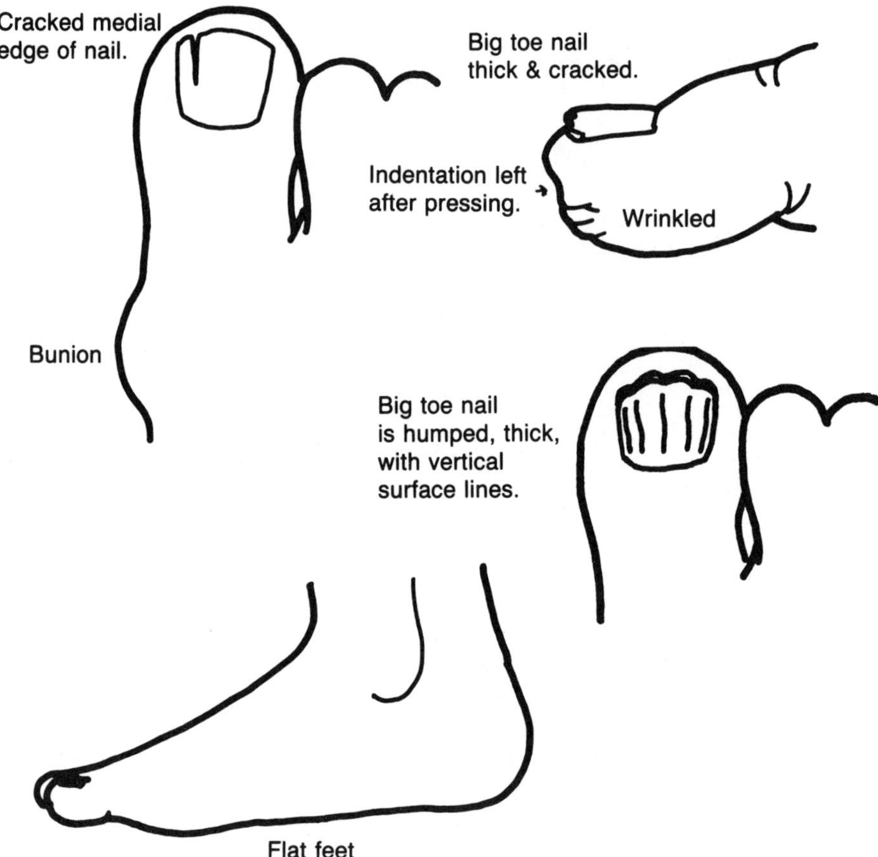
Cracked medial edge of nail.
Big toe nail thick & cracked.
Indentation left after pressing.
Wrinkled
Bunion
Big toe nail is humped, thick, with vertical surface lines.
Flat feet

Figure 41

Tension or tightness between the shoulder blades is a sign of tai yin problems; thus the lungs and not necessarily the spleen may be implicated. Careful differentiation is required. When a tense or swollen lower abdomen is present, indicating spleen deficiency, there is often a tightness and swelling that makes noises when pressed. Sores on or behind the lips generally indicate a spleen deficiency in association with a stomach excess. The patient who is hungry and is unable to eat will feel weak and lack energy, a hypoglycemic reaction. This is common in spleen deficient conditions. In more advanced stages it may become a diabetic condition, a severe spleen deficiency. Look for the callus on the inside of the left big toe, this is often present.

Feeling sleepy after eating is a good indication of a spleen and kidney deficiency, often accompanying a slight stomach excess. This condition is a typical ten stem disharmony. Within the earth element the yin aspect, spleen, is deficient; the yang aspect, stomach, is slightly excess. This imbalance transmits in the earth-water (controlling) relationship, where earth yang, stomach, and water yin, kidney, interact resulting in a kidney deficiency.[5]

Liver Deficiency

Palpation

Tension, tightness, pressure pain, puffiness and resistance below the ribs on the right side, especially around right ST-19, LV-13 and LV-14, are liver deficiency signals. Here, interpret LV-14 as directly below the ribs on a vertical line below the nipple. Pressure pain, tightness, tension and pulsing to the left of the navel are also frequent liver deficiency signals. Examine closely the area between and just above left ST-25 to left ST-27 (sometimes spread slightly medial of the stomach line, lateral towards the spleen meridian). Pressure pain on left LV-9, often with pressure pain on left LV-8 and sometimes LV-3, and pressure pain and tension on and around the right shoulder blade are also indicative of liver deficiency.

Accompanying Signs

Stiff shoulders, especially the right shoulder;
Dislike of wind or dryness;
Chronic headaches;
Weak legs, particularly the left leg;
Oversensitivity;
Heaviness of the legs;
Legs that easily become edematous, especially the left leg;
Fainting easily;
Dizziness;
Cold feet;
Uncomfortable feeling below the ribs, specially the right side;
Myopia;
Muscles easily become tense, tight, contracted;
Strained back;
Asthma.

The liver deficient person will be more susceptible to acute back problems or more likely to have a history of acute back problems. However, recurrent back problems should also cue us to check for a yin wei mai—chong mai condition. The patient may be emotional; they can become angry easily and frequently, just as easily forgetting the cause of their anger. Often after getting angry, the liver deficient person feels tired. Anger that results from a deficient liver condition is distinguished by frequent occurrence and short duration. Excess liver anger, which is rare, is stronger, more intense and long lived. Often the liver excess person remains angry for a long time.

It is interesting to note that almost all asthmatic patients take some medication. Whether the asthma was originally from a deficient liver condition, or the deficiency developed from the medication, most asthmatics manifest liver deficiency. Medications **always** create liver deficiency, **never** liver excess. It is also common to find a large intestine excess, in association with a liver deficiency. In asthmatics this may be accompanied by a lung deficiency, a common ten stem relationship. Within the metal element, if the yang aspect (large intestine) becomes excess, both the yin component (lungs) and the yin component of the wood element (liver) will be deficient. In these cases, large intestine points such as LI-4 and LI-10 can become very reactive, especially on the right side. If after cupping around BL-17, BL-18 and below the ribs on the right side, the skin turns a uniform light pink, this can be a sign of liver deficiency. This response is often found in patients who are taking many medications. A redder color is healthier.

Toe and eye changes:

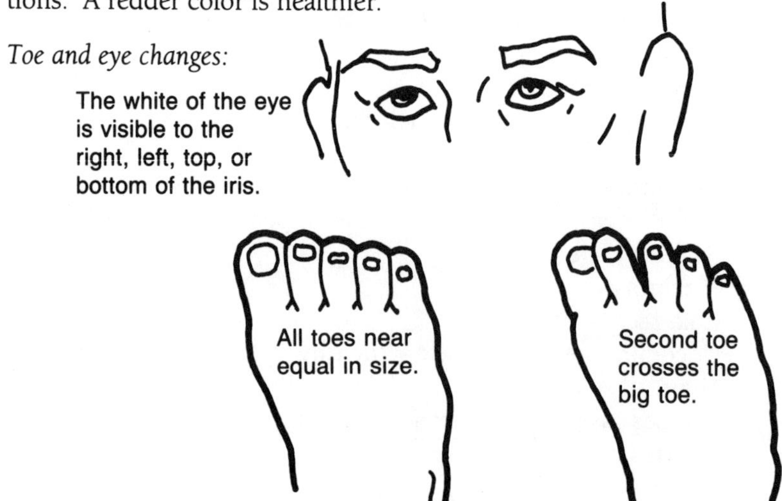
The white of the eye is visible to the right, left, top, or bottom of the iris.
All toes near equal in size.
Second toe crosses the big toe.

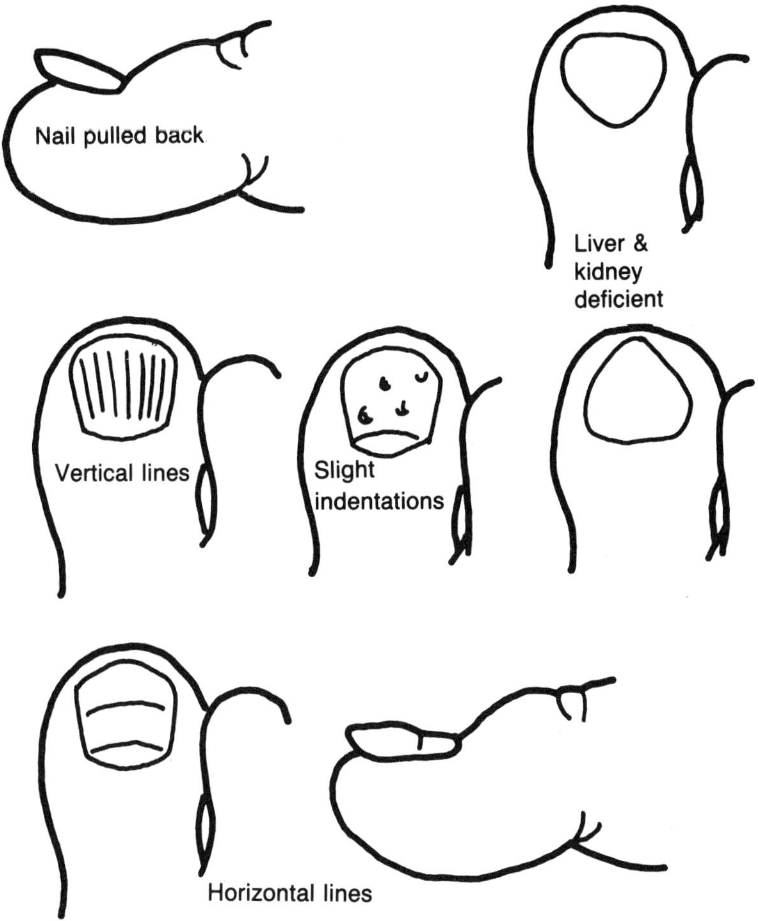

Figure 42

Lung Deficiency

Palpation

Lung deficient patients often evidence pressure pain, tension, tightness and pulsing to the right of the navel, generally around right ST-25 to ST-26. Pressure pain, tension and tightness at a point that is on a line from the navel to the superior anterior corner of the right iliac crest, one third of the distance from the navel to the crest, is also a lung deficiency indication. Pressure pain, tension on LU-1, especially right LU-1, and pressure pain or looseness and weakness on LU-9, especially right LU-9, is also a reliable sign. Pressure pain on LU-6 (three divisions below LU-5) is present in acute lung conditions. When a lung deficient patient catches cold the rectus abdominis muscle on the right side often becomes tense with reaction on right ST-27.

Accompanying Signs

Catches cold easily;
Tension between the shoulder blades;
Poor posture;
Sleeps in a fetal or shrimp posture;
Difficulty breathing deeply;
Skin becomes dry;
Vascular spider on the cheeks.

Remember this tension between the shoulders is also a tai yin sign and could also be spleen related. The posture to keep in mind displays the shoulders forward, the person slouching. The back might be slightly hunched, the spine curved forward, especially from GV-12, which can become sensitive. Where there are breathing difficulties, breathing is generally shallow. The person might inhale strongly, yet exhale in a short shallow breath like an asthmatic. In lung deficient, large intestine excess conditions there will often be constipation or hemorrhoids. Children who exhibit lung deficiency tend to be quiet, not to talk much and to be inactive.

Nail changes:

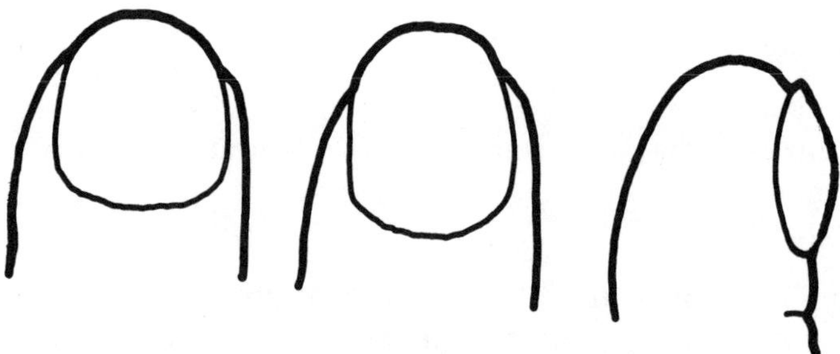

The nails, particularly of the thumb, are unusually large, or spoon-shaped.

Figure 43

Kidney Deficiency

The kidney is always seen as becoming deficient and never excess.

Palpation

Pulsing below the navel;
Pulsing on CV-9;
Weakness, flaccidity, coolness below the navel;
Tightness below the navel;
Abdomen swollen above and indented below the navel;
Tightness along the center line below the navel;
Pressure pain on KI-16;
Pressure pain, weakness, puffiness around KI-2.

Pulsing on CV-9 also relates to spleen deficiency. In both of the reactions below the navel a main feature when the patient is kidney deficient is a lack of elasticity.

Accompanying signs

Bones break easily;
Ankles sprain easily;
Body easily becomes puffy or edematous;
Dental caries;
Cold in the back or lower areas of the body;
Bleeding gums;
Tinnitus;
Runny nose that stops with application of heat to the body;
Hair falls out easily;
Easily frightened;
Forgetful.

If the patient's feet are disproportionately skinny, thin and weak, with a dry, lustreless skin surface, this may be a sign of prenatal kidney deficiency.

Nail and Foot Signs:

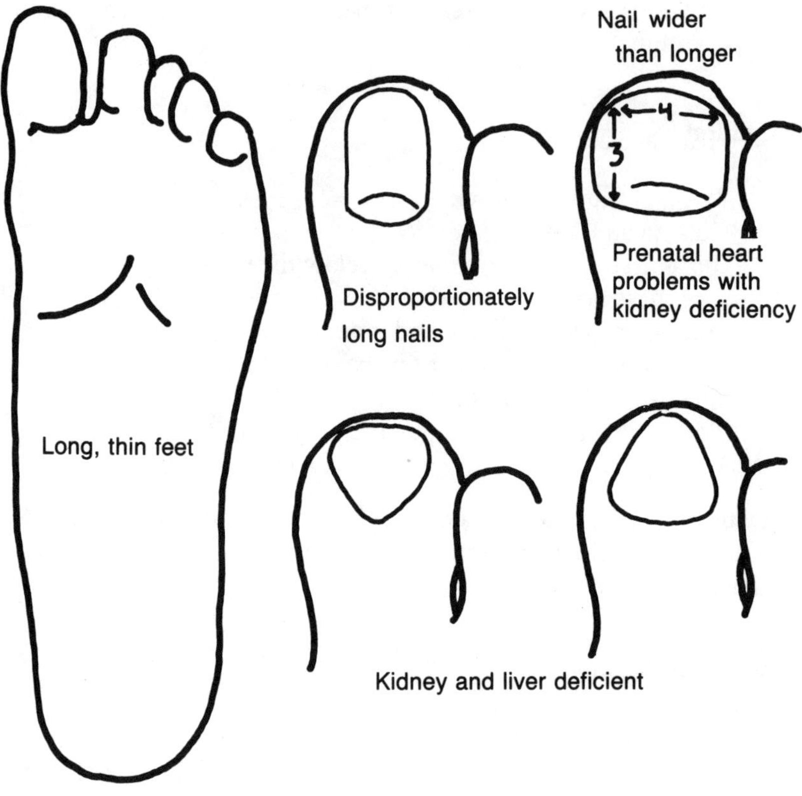

Figure 44

Heart Problems

Because the heart stores the shen and is the "emperor," it never becomes deficient, as this results in death. When we see patients with heart problems, they are usually of an excess nature, and are related to weakness of the kidneys. A worker in the emergency room of a hospital might see heart deficient patients, but fewer acupuncturists treat patients with this condition.

Palpation

Pulsing in the upper abdomen on the center line;
Upper back tight, knotted or tense;
Pressure pain, tension, tightness directly below the sternum;
Pressure pain on PC-4;
Heart palpitations;
Heart attacks.

The center line abdominal pulsing will generally be found in the CV-12 to CV-15 area. This sign is often found in neurotic patients. Where heart deficiency is indicated, the upper back near BL-38, and no other area, will feel tight, knotted or tense. Pressure pain on PC-4 (three divisions below PC-3) will be found with acute heart problems.

Accompanying Signs

The abdomen will be fuller above than below. Generally the overall shape of the normal abdomen is larger above the pelvis and relatively narrower below the sternum. However, in patients with heart problems the abdomen can be shaped such that the area below the sternum is wider and narrows as it descends to the pelvic region. If the area around ming tang (between the eyebrows) is red, the patient currently has a heart problem. If the area is dark red, it is a chronic heart problem. If there are several tiny red spots in this area, the condition is dangerous. Sometimes there will be tiny white spots in this area; this too is a dangerous sign, particularly if the area is generally colored a dark red.

To help prevent heart attacks, it is important to teach the patient abdominal breathing and clenching of the muscles of the anus. They should practice this every day.

Nail Signs:

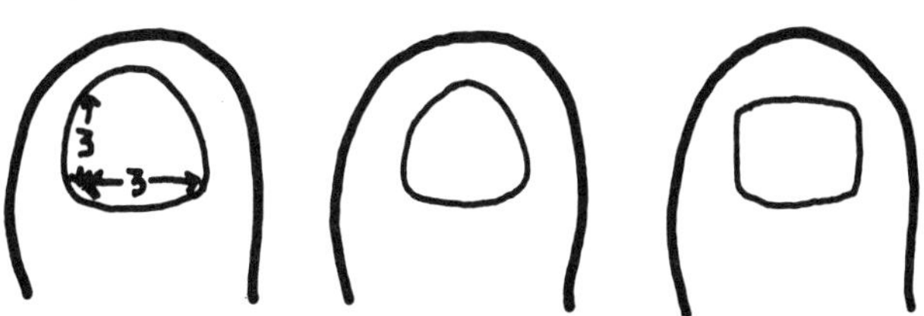

Figure 45 The nails are relatively small.

Treatment Principles

Follow the instructions given in the previous chapter. When using the pointer machine, remember that the north magnet is placed either on the most reactive point in the reflective area on the knees and back or on the most affected area or point. The south magnet is placed on a point that is useful for the diagnosed deficient condition.

Appendix Two
Electromagnetic
Treatment of Scars

Electromagnetic treatments may be effective for treating pathologies caused by the scarring that results from traumatic injury or surgical procedures.[6] Often we treat patients who have had an injury or surgery that leaves a scar. These scars can become the source of other problems by weakening and obstructing the flow of energy through the meridians. The obstruction is generally the result of the formation of scar tissues in the superficial and deeper tissues that distorts the normal tissues and the energy flow through them. In most cases where the scar is pathological, it will traverse one or more meridians. The topological relationships of each scar will be different from person to person, depending on the natural strengths, weaknesses and predispositions of the patient. Different symptoms can result from scars in the same place. Thus, even for scars that appear identical, different therapeutic principles or approaches may be required.

Often scars are not pathological. Sometimes, however, it will be obvious when a disorder is present. For example, a female patient told us that since breast surgery she had experienced pain in the chest or breast that occurred in damp weather, an obvious cue for scar treatment. Also, a patient might describe a pulling pain that seems to originate from the scar, or knee pain that relates to a scar from knee surgery. Even if the trauma or surgery occurred many years previous, such relationships should indicate scar therapy. There are other cases where the association of the scar to a particular problem is less obvious. The diagnosis of these conditions may generally be ascertained only by palpation and experimental treatment of the scar. If you find sharp pressure pain on one or more points along the scar or a feeling of discomfort, causing radiating sensations when pressed, or even just unpleasant sensations, scar therapy is indicated. The reactive points are the points to treat.

Generally, treat scars by placing the (N)$^{-3000}$ on the most reactive point on the scar and the (S)$^{-3000}$ further down the meridian on the scar on a reactive point. The (S)$^{-3000}$ may also be placed further down the meridian below the scar, perhaps one to three inches below, or much further down the meridian. For example, consider the case of pain around the eyebrows where there is a traumatic scar that runs roughly along the bladder meridian extending about one inch upward from BL-2. First, palpate the scar; find the most reactive point and place the (N)$^{-3000}$ here. If there is another reactive point higher on the scar, place the (S)$^{-3000}$ there. If your initial palpation does not locate a reactive point on the scar itself, begin by palpating above the scar. Then apply the pointer machine as previously described. If this treatment does not change the reaction after a three to five minutes, try palpating the meridian close to the scar, about one to three inches from the scar. If you locate a reactive point, place the (S)$^{-3000}$ on it. If after a few minutes of treatment there is still no change of the reactivity found, or if there is no reactive point above the scar, palpate further down the bladder meridian. Begin far from the eyes, around BL-60 or BL-62. If a point in this area is reactive, place the (S)$^{-3000}$ on the point. Generally one of these three procedures will ameliorate the presenting problem.

For pain in the right breast with a surgical scar on the lateral edge of the breast, palpate the scar to find the most reactive point; place the (N)$^{-3000}$ on the point. If there is another reactive point on the scar, place the (S)$^{-3000}$ on that point. Alternately, use a reactive point one to three inches below the scar. However, if after checking no changes in point reactions or no reactive points can be found, then palpate distally for the location of the initial placement of the (S)$^{-3000}$. Usually, the breasts are related to the stomach meridians that run through them. This would indicate using a reactive stomach meridian point for the location of the (S)$^{-3000}$. However, if treatment of a distal stomach point does not elicit good results, treatment of distal spleen points (the associated or coupled meridian) so as to tonify the spleen would be indicated. Often, SP-3 or SP-6 are the best points to use.

Note that this treatment follows the principle of treating along the pathway of the meridian, or extending treatment to two contiguous meridians, in this case the stomach and spleen. The example treatment further utilizes tonification of a deficient meridian. If the yang meridian, the stomach, is obstructed, it becomes excess, causing a relative deficiency of the spleen meridian. Thus, if the spleen is **the** deficient meridian, the treatment will be particularly effective. In effect, the electromagnetic application would treat two conditions at once, both releasing the stress at the scar and tonifying the primary deficiency.

Appendix Three Electromagnetic Zone Therapy

Occasionally, following all your usual treatment procedures still will not yield satisfactory results. In these cases, a fourth style of pointer machine use may be helpful. This style utilizes the ideas and treatment points of Dr. Zhang Xin Shu, from his book *Wan Ke Zhen, Wrist Ankle Acupuncture.*[7] Dr. Zhang Xin Shu discovered six points on each wrist and above each ankle that correlated with zones on the body. These points and zones are coupled, one upper to one lower zone. Thus, there are six zones each with an upper and lower treatment point. The upper points, "upper 1 to 6" are located at a level two finger widths above the wrist. The lower points, "lower 1 to 6" are located three finger widths above the tip of the ankles. The six zones are somewhat similar to the coupled meridians in the shao yin, tai yang, jue yin pairs, though obviously different in several respects. The upper points control their correspondent zones above the diaphragm and the lower points control the zones below the diaphragm.[8]

Dr. Shu selects from these points and treats them with needles inserted subcutaneously and gently, laterally one to one and a half inches, retaining the needles for thirty minutes. We recommend treating the same points with the pointer machine techniques previously described. We have regularly obtained excellent clinical results by using these points conjunctively with local treatments or with treatments of the reactive knee and lower back areas described in the previous chapter. Points may be selected according to two principles. If the patient's problem clearly lies on a zone, above or below the diaphragm, the appropriate upper or lower associated point should be palpated. Next, if the patient's problems match the symptoms associated with a zone, palpate the associated treatment point. In either case, if the appropriate point is reactive it may be treated. However, if the associated point is not reactive, the zone treatments are not indicated.

Treatment of these points can be helpful for stubborn conditions of the knee and sacral areas. Lower 3, 4 and 6, targeting the medial and lateral eye of the knee areas, and the edges of the sacrum, are particularly useful. For example, if you diagnose a patient with sciatica as having a yang wei—dai mai problem, you would treat SI-3 and left TW-5 with N^{600}, BL-62 and right GB-41 (because the right leg was longer) with S^{600}; then $(N)^{-6000}$ on the left lateral superior corner of the sacrum and $(S)^{-3000}$ on the lateral eye of the left knee (because both were reactive). However, if this treatment only adjusted the legs slightly and produced no decrease in the reaction at the indicative knee area, you would consider using the zone points. In this example Lower 4 would be indicated to eliminate the knee reaction.

If the Lower 4 point were sore, you could try placing the $(N)^{-3000}$ on the knee area and the $(S)^{-3000}$ on left Lower 4. If this combination works, not only will the knee area reaction decrease, but the legs will also adjust. Generally, the first placement of the pointer machine would require three to four minutes before checking and switching if needed, and the second placement would require another three to four minutes before success was obtained. Thus, if we are clear in logic and procedure we can elicit favorable results in only ten to fifteen minutes. The magnets are then left on for a total of twenty minutes.

Of course, if this treatment produced no decrease of the knee area reaction, we would consider the condition of the elements and meridians to see if the source of the problem were an active deficiency requiring treatment. It is important to consider all potential conditions. Yet, after following all the recommended procedures, there are patients with pain problems that are extremely resistant. These stubborn pain patients require a "painkilling" treatment. Palpation to determine if the appropriate points are reactive is the key for effective treatment of stubborn pain in the limbs.

This style utilizes points that are located topologically opposite to each other, *e.g.*, PC-6 and TW-5, or SP-10 and ST-33. In China these points are treated with deep needling, what is called "through and through acupuncture." For instance, TW-5 is needled through to PC-6, or LI-4 to SI-3.[9] In Japan, moxa treatments of points similarly topologically located have developed, where tiny moxa is burnt on TW-5 and PC-6 or SP-10 and ST-33.[10] On occasion, according to the indications for each of these pairs of points, the $(N)^{-3000}$ and $(S)^{-3000}$ can be used effectively to replace deep needling or double moxa. Though seldom used, it can be helpful. Common combinations are:

Point Pair		Problem Area
TW-5	PC-6	wrist, hand problems
TW-4	PC-7	wrist problems
LI-4	SI-3	hand problems
ST-33	SP-10	knee problems
GB-34	SP-9	knee problems
GB-35	LV-6	leg problems
GB-39	SP-6	leg, gynecologic and bladder problems

To use these point combinations it is necessary to differentiate the side of the limb that is most affected. The (N)-3000 should go on that side and the (S)-3000 on the opposite. Thus, for someone with a wrist problem, if the problem lies more on the back of the hand or wrist, the (N)-3000 should go on TW-4 or TW-5 and the (S)-3000 on PC-7 or PC-6 (depending on the points that were most reactive).

Notes

[1] The following practitioners work has been used in the preparation of this essay:

Sorei Yanagiya, *Kanmei Humon Shinsatsu Ho*; Denmei Shudo, *Keiraku Chiryo no Susume*; Shohaku Honma, *Keiraku Chiryo Kuowa*; Sodo Okabe, *Shinkyu Keiraku Chiryo*; Tsugio Nagatomo, *Nagatomo M.P. Shinkyu Kuowa Hachiju Hachisyu*; Yoshio Manaka, from notes, lectures and his many publications.

[2] See *Five Elements and Ten Stems,* pp. 111-115.

[3] See *Hara: Reflections on the Sea.*

[4] For general discussions of diagnosis, diagnostic signs and process, see *Five Elements and Ten Stems,* pp. 89-129, and *Hara: Reflections on the Sea.*

[5] See *Five Elements and Ten Stems,* pp. 27-32 and 51-64 for more discussion.

[6] Dr. Chen Zhi reports good success with patients in treating reactive scars.

[7] *Wan Ke Zhen, Wrist Ankle Acupuncture,* has been translated into Japanese by Mitsutane Sugi and published by Ido no Nippon Sha, 1979.

[8] The series of symptoms that Dr. Shu found associated with each of these zones are listed in Chapter 4.

[9] *Cf. Kuai Su Zhen Ci Liao Fa.*

[10] *Cf.* Isaburo Fukaya, *Fukaya Kyu Ho.*

Bibliography

Citations in the text or in footnotes with page references refer to the specific editions texts listed in the bibliography. Thus, *Su Wen,* Chapter 60, p. 319, refers to the *Huang Di Nei Jing Su Wen* published by the People's Hygiene Publishing company, first edition, 1978. Although this text arose from a larger research project, *Hara Diagnosis,* the bibliography details only the specific citations in this text. The ideas presented draw on many other works; references may be found in the larger text. This is particularly true of the theoretical and scientific models.

Medical Bibliography

Akabane, K. 皮内針法
Hinaishin Ho {Methods of hinaishin}. Yokosuka: Ido No Nippon Sha, 1964.

Bensky, D., and O'Connor, J.
Acupuncture, A Comprehensive Text. Chicago: Eastland Press, 1981.

Chen Zhi. 磁療法
Ci Liao Fa {Methods of magnet treatment}. Hunan: Science and Technology Publishing Co, 1979.

Dou Jie. 針経指南
Zhen Jing Zhi Nan {Acupuncture text, south pointer}. Circa 1295. From *Zhen Jiu Si Shu* {Acupuncture and moxibustion four books}. Compiled circa 1311. Beijing: People's Hygiene Publishing Company, 1983.

Fukaya, Isaburo. 深谷灸法
Fukaya Kyu Ho {Fukaya's moxa treatment style}. Tokyo: Shizensha, 1980.

Gao Wu. 鍼灸聚英
Zhen Jiu Ju Ying {Gathering of eminent acupuncturists}. 1529. Shanghai: Shanghai Science and Technology Publishing Company, 1961.

Honma, Shohaku. 経絡治療講話
Keiraku Chiryo Kuowa {Lectures on five element treatment}. Yokosuka: Ido No Nippon Sha, 1947.

__________. 鍼灸病証学
Shinkyu Byosho Gaku {Diseases and configurations in the study of acupuncture and moxibustion}. Yokosuka: Ido No Nippon Sha, 1943.

Hua Shou. 十四経発揮
Shi Si Jing Fa Hui {Elucidation of the fourteen meridians}. 1341. Yokosuka: Ido No Nippon Sha, 1946.

黄帝内經靈樞
Huang Di Nei Jing Ling Shu {*Ling Shu*}. Circa 100-300 BC. From 黄帝内經靈樞譯解
Huang Di Nei Jing Ling Shu Yi Jie {Yellow Emperor Nei Jing Ling Shu Explanatory Text}. 2nd. ed. Taipei: Chinese Republic Publishing Company, 1978.

黄帝内經素問
Huang Di Nei Jing Su Wen {*Su Wen*}. Beijing: People's Hygiene Publishing Company, 1978.

Huang Fu Mi. 針灸甲乙経
Zhen Jiu Jia Yi Jing {Systematic classic of acupuncture and moxibustion}. 282. Quoted *Nei Jing Jie Po Sheng Li Xue*, pp. 117 and 143.

Ito, Osamu. 11円で胃カイヨウは治る
Juichien de Ikayio ga Naoru {Treatment of stomach ulcers using eleven yen}. Tokyo: Jitsu Gyo No Nippon Sha, 1981.

__________.
"Magnetic Electric Acupuncture Without Needles (PIA Therapy)." Seminar handbook, n.d.

金匱要略方論
Jinkui Yaolue Fanglun {Prescriptions from the golden chamber}. Circa 220. Quoted from *Qi Jing Ba Mai Kao*, vol. 1, p. 23.

快速針刺療法
Kuai Su Zhen Ci Liao Fa. Shen Yang: Chinese Peoples Liberation Army Air Force Hospital, 1969.

Li Shi Zhen. 奇經八脈攷
Qi Jing Ba Mai Kao {An examination of the eight extraordinary vessels}. Circa 1570. Found in the *Tu Zhu Nan Jing Mai Jue* (*q.v.*)

Manaka, Yoshio, MD, PhD. 医家のための鍼術入門講座
Ika no Tameno Shinjutsu Nyumon Kuoza {Introductory lectures on acupuncture for medical doctors}. 2nd. ed. Tokyo: Ido No Nippon Sha, 1980.

__________.
"Kenkyu ni Oyoshita Jiki Kotoni sono Keiketsu Sessyoku Koka ni Tsuite." {Research into the effects of magnets and specifically the effects on certain acupoints}. Lecture pamphlet, n.d.

__________. 針灸の理論と考え方
Shinkyu no Riron to Kangaekata 2nd. ed. {Thoughts and theory of acupuncture and moxibustion}. Osaka: Sogen Igaku Sha, 1980.

Nagatomo, Tsugio. 長友・MP鍼灸講話八十八輯
Nagatomo M.P. Shinkyu Kuowa Hachiju Hachisyu {Mr. Nagatomo's 88 lectures on the minus-plus needle therapy}. Kyoto: Shinkyu Shinkuokai Sha, 1976.

難經
Nan Jing {Classic of difficulties}. Circa 100 BC - 100 AD. Found in *Tu Zhu Nan Jing Mai Jue (q.v.)*

Nan Jing Medical School. 針灸学
Zhen Jiu Xue {Acupuncture and moxibustion studies} Shanghai: Shanghai Science and Technology Publishing Company, 1979.

内經解剖生理学
Nei Jing Jie Po Sheng Li Xue {Anatomy and Physiology of the Nei Jing}. 2nd. ed. Taiwan: National Chinese Medical Herb Research Center Publishing Company, 1977.

Okabe, Sodo. 鍼灸経絡治療
Shinkyu keiraku chiryo {Acupuncture and moxibustion five elements treatments}. Tokyo: Seki Bundo Sha, 1974.

Shudo, Denmei. 経絡治療のすすめ
Keiraku Chiryo no Susume {Recommendations for five element treatments}. Yokosuka: Ido No Nippon Sha, 1984.

So, James Tin Yau.
Book of Acupuncture Points. Brookline: Paradigm Publications, 1985.

Sugiyama, Waichi. 杉山流三部書
Sugiyama Ryu Sanbusho. {Sugiyama's style of treatment in three parts}. 2nd. ed. Circa 1700. Yokosuka: Ido No Nippon Sha, 1978.

圖註難経脈訣
Tu Zhu Nan Jing Mai Jue {Art of nan jing pulses, with illustrations}. 2nd. ed. Taiwan: Shui Cheng Shu Ju Publishing Company, 1970.

Wan Wei Yi. 銅人腧穴鍼灸図経
Tongren Shu Xue Zhen Jiu Tu Jing {Bronze statue textbook} 1027. Compiled by Masao Maruyama. Tokyo: Seiko Bundo Publishing Company, 1970.

Wang Shu He. 脈經
Mai Jing {Classic of the pulse}. Circa 300 AD. 2nd. ed. Taiwan: Shang Wu Yin Shu Publishing Company, 1963.

__________.
{Commentary on the Nan Jing}. Circa 300 AD. Found in *Tu Zhu Nan Jing Mai Jue* (*q.v.*)

Xu Feng. 鍼灸大全
Zhen Jiu Da Quan {Complete textbook of acupuncture and moxibustion}. 1437. From *Bi Chao Zhen Jiu Da Quan*. Circa 1600. Taiwan: Han Wu Publishing Company, 1974.

Xu Xi Nien. 子午針灸療法
Zi Wu Zhen Jiu Liao Fa {Calendrical (branch 1, branch 7) acupuncture moxibustion treatments}. Hong Kong: Nan Guang Publishing Co, n.d.

Yanagiya, Sorei. 簡明不問診察法
Kanmei Humon Shinsatsu Ho {Diagnosis without asking} 2nd ed. Tokyo: Ishiyama Shinkyu Igaku Publishing Company, 1976.

Yang Ji Zhou. 針灸大成
Zhen Jiu Da Cheng {Compendium of acupuncture and moxibustion} 1601. Taiwan: Hong Ye Shu Ju Publishing Company, 1976.

Yang Shang San. 黄帝内經太素
Huang Di Nei Jing Tai Su {*Tai Su*}. Circa 610. Beijing: People's Hygiene Publishing Company, 1965.

Zhang Jie Bing. 類經
Lei Jing {Classic of categories}. 1624. Beijing: People's Hygiene Publishing Company, 1965.

Zhang Xin Shu. 足根針
Wan Ke Zhen {Wrist ankle acupuncture}. Translated by Matsutane Sugi. Yokosuka: Ido No Nippon Sha, 1979.

針灸經外奇穴图譜
Zhen Jiu Jing Wai Qi Xue Tu Du {Acupuncture and moxibustion non-meridian extra point atlas}. Shanxi: Hygiene Publishing Co., 1963.

Reference and non-medical bibliography

Bohm, David. *Wholeness and the Implicate Order.* London: Ark paperbacks, 1980.

諸橋大漢和辞典
Daikanwa Jiten {Morohashi encyclopedic dictionary of classical Chinese} Tokyo: Daishukan Sha, 1959.

Fujido, Akiyasu. 藤堂漢和大字典
Gakuken Kanwadaijiten {Fujido's etymological dictionary} Tokyo: Gakushu Kenkyu Sha, 1978.

淮南子
Huai Nan Zi {Book of master huai nan}. Circa 122 BC. With commentary by Haruki Kusuyama. Tokyo: Meiji Syoin Sha, 1979.

簡明中医辞典
Jing Ming Zhong Yi Ci Dian {Explanatory dictionary of Chinese medicine}. Hong Kong: Joint Publishing Company, 1979.

Kato, Joken, and Yamada, Katsuni. 角川字源辞典
Kadokawa Jigenjiten. {Kadokawa etymological dictionary}. Tokyo: Kadokawa Publishing Company, 1972.

列子
Lie Zi {Book of Master Lie}. Circa 500-100 BC. Quoted from *Daikanwa Jiten* {Morohashi encyclopedic dictionary}.

Maspero, Henri. *Taoism and Chinese religion.* Amherst: University of Massachusetts Press, 1981.

Nakagawa, Kyoichi.
"Magnetic field deficiency syndrome and magnetic treatment. *Japan Medical Journal* 2745 (December 1975).

Needham, Joseph. *Science and Civilization in China.* vol. 4, part 1. Cambridge: Cambridge University Press, 1962.

Wilber, Ken, ed. *The Holographic Paradigm and other Paradoxes.* Boulder: Shambhala Publications, 1982.

老子荘子
Zhuang Zi {Book of Master Zhuang}. Circa 300 BC. Taken from Ogawa, Harukai. *Lao Zi, Zhuang Zi.* Tokyo: Chuo Koron Sha, 1978.

Index

This index is divided into three sections. The first is a general index of reference terms as used through-out the text. The second section, beginning on page 277 and continuing to page 291, is all of the symptom, sign and energetic concepts used in the treatment sections and the actions and effects comparisons. Finally, begining on page 291, the points themselves are indexed.

Symptom Index

□ *Q* □

□ *R* □

□ S □

□ *Y* □

Point Index

The following codes are used:
D = Classic & *Da Cheng*
T = Theoretical discussion
M = Modern Treatments
C = Comparative effects